ACE Inhibition
after
Myocardial Infarction

The authors wish to thank Sara Churchill and Dr Alistair Hall for their invaluable help in the preparation of this book.

ACE Inhibition

after

Myocardial Infarction

L B Tan

Department of Cardiology
University of Leeds
Leeds, UK

S G Ball

Department of Cardiovascular Studies
University of Leeds
Leeds, UK

SCIENCE PRESS

British Cataloguing-in-Publication Data.
A catalogue record for this book is available from the British Library.

ISBN: 1-85873-015-5

This copy of *ACE Inhibition after Myocardial Infarction* is given as a service to medicine by Hoechst. Sponsorship of this copy does not imply the sponsor's agreement or otherwise with the views expressed herein.

Although every effort has been made to ensure that drug doses and other information are presented accurately in this publication, the ultimate responsibility rests with the prescribing physician. Neither the publishers nor the authors can be held responsible for errors or for any consequences arising from the use of information contained herein. Any product mentioned in this publication should be used in accordance with the prescribing information prepared by the manufacturers. No claims or endorsements are made for any drug or compound at present under clinical investigation.

Project development editor: Sara Churchill
Project editor: Kathryn Orchard
Illustrators: Paul Bernson and Stuart Molloy
Typesetter: Neil Morris
Production: Christina Quigley
Printed in Spain

Cover illustration: Transverse section of human heart to show expansion of an anterior infarction. Courtesy of MJ Davies.

Contents

Abbreviations

ACE	angiotensin converting enzyme
AIRE	Acute Infarction Ramipril Efficacy [Study]
BCT	brachiocephalic trunk
CATS	Captopril and Thrombolysis Study
CHD	coronary heart disease
CONSENSUS	Cooperative North Scandinavian Enalapril Survival Study
GISSI	Gruppo Italiano per lo Studio della Sopravvivenza nell'Infarto Miocardio
ISIS	International Studies of Infarct Survival
LIVCA	left interventricular coronary artery
LVH	left ventricular hypertrophy
PDGF	platelet-derived growth factor
PTCA	percutaneous transluminal coronary angioplasty
RAS	renin–angiotensin system
SAVE	Survival and Ventricular Enlargement [Study]
SK	streptokinase
SMILE	Survival of Myocardial Infarction Long-term Evaluation
SOLVD	Studies of Left Ventricular Dysfunction
SPECT	single photon emission computed tomography
TIMI	Thrombolysis in Myocardial Infarction [Study]
tPA	tissue-type plasminogen activator
TRACE	[The] Trandolapril Cardiac Evaluation [Study]

1

Myocardial infarction: an introduction

Myocardial infarction can be seen as part of a continuum of pathological events initiated by coronary arterial atherosclerosis. It is the underlying event in the majority of deaths from cardiovascular disease in Western society. In future it might be possible to prevent or regress coronary atherosclerosis, thus obviating the occurrence of myocardial infarction. Until then, however, our coronary-care units are still filled daily with patients who have suffered a myocardial infarction. In the UK alone each year, 170 000 deaths are attributed to myocardial infarction, with some 330 000 infarctions. A minority of patients benefit from recanalization of the occluded arteries by pharmacological or interventional means, thereby aborting or limiting the infarction. The major complications of infarction, arrhythmias and heart failure are the common causes of death after an infarction. The extent to which the myocardium is damaged by the initiating event is an important determinant of prognosis.

Vascular remodelling leading to myocardial infarction

Atherosclerosis is a chronic, progressive, multifocal intimal disease usually characterized by the presence of a raised plaque with a core containing lipids, complex carbohydrates, blood and blood products, and a fibrous outer coat (Fig. 1.1) [1]. Plaques are often calcified, and the degree of calcification appears to be related to the severity of stenosis and the age of the individual [2].

Nearly all cases of acute myocardial infarction occur in patients with pre-existing coronary atherosclerosis. The assumption that atherosclerosis of the coronary arteries is the prerequisite for myocardial infarction is based on detailed post-mortem studies of patients dying from cardiac and non-cardiac causes, and coronary angiography and angioscopy of cardiac patients [3–8]. It is supported by the observation that the mean number of atherosclerotic plaques in people dying of non-cardiac causes correlates with the frequency of death from ischaemic heart disease in the same population [9].

Characteristics of a typical atherosclerotic plaque

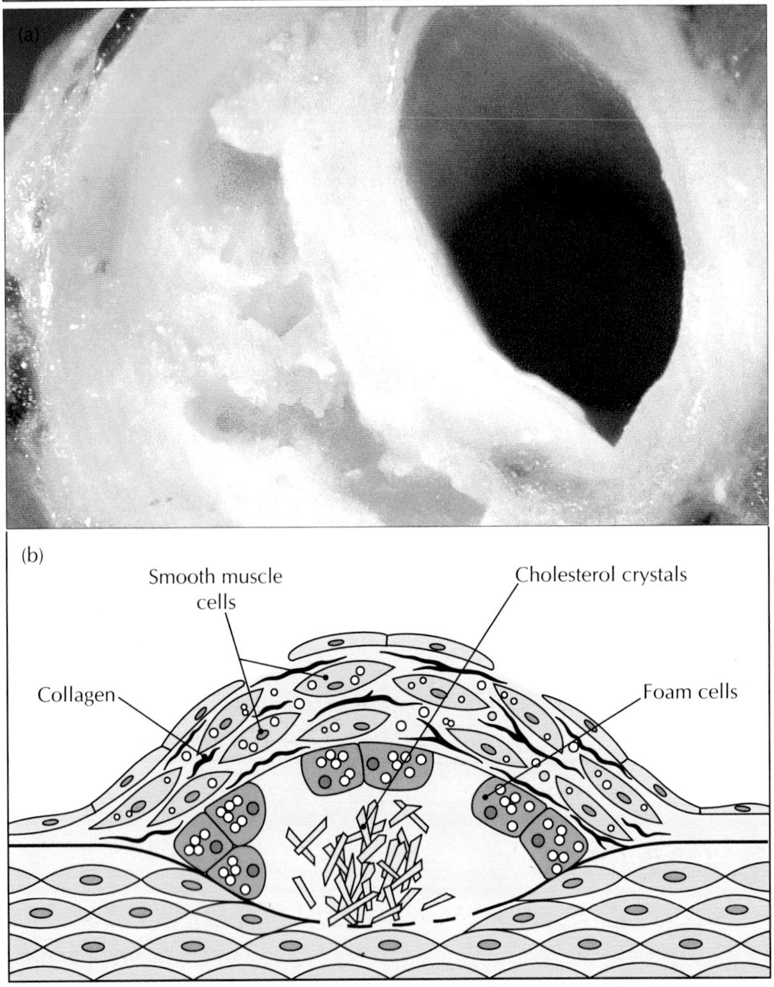

Fig. 1.1. (a) Transverse section of human coronary artery to show a large lipid-rich advanced plaque. The plaque has a large lipid core, which is soft and has begun to break down, leaving a cavity in the plaque. The lipid core is separated from the lumen by a thick cap of fibrous tissue. Courtesy of MJ Davies. (b) Diagrammatic representation of an atheromatous plaque showing the outer cap containing collagen and smooth muscle cells and inner core containing foam cells and extracellular crystals. Adapted by permission [56].

The gross pattern of events is thought to be as follows: an atheromatous plaque causes a narrowing of the coronary artery lumen leading to myocardial ischaemia, thrombosis and subsequent infarction (Fig. 1.2). Many atheromatous plaques, however, extend externally into the artery wall rather than into the lumen. Because such lesions do not impede blood flow, they may not cause symptoms and are not apparent on angiography [10]. This may explain why thromboses leading to myocardial infarction often occur in regions that appear angiographically to be free of atheroma or to have minimal lesions [11]. Indeed, the majority of fatal myocardial infarctions may result from thrombosis occurring on minimal lesions. It also suggests that the primary catastrophic event is not the ischaemia resulting from occlusion of the coronary artery but the plaque rupture leading to coronary thrombosis. The degree and location of the infarct depend

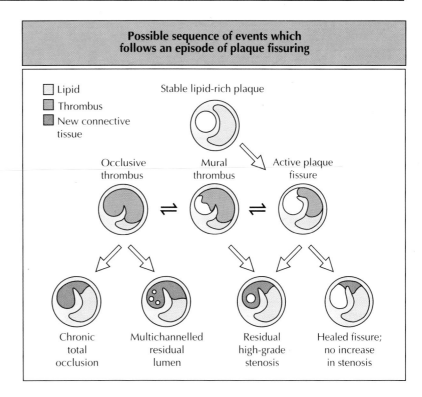

Possible sequence of events which follows an episode of plaque fissuring

☐ Lipid
☐ Thrombus
☐ New connective tissue

Stable lipid-rich plaque

Occlusive thrombus — Mural thrombus — Active plaque fissure

Chronic total occlusion — Multichannelled residual lumen — Residual high-grade stenosis — Healed fissure; no increase in stenosis

Fig. 1.2. Diagrammatic representation of the sequence of events in plaque fissuring (deep intimal injury) and the range of possible long-term results. Adapted by permission [57].

on which coronary artery is occluded, and on the adequacy, or otherwise, of the collateral blood supply to the region beyond the stenosis [12].

Plaque formation

Plaque formation in the coronary circulation is characterized by a long asymptomatic phase that begins in early childhood. In human babies, vascular smooth muscle proliferation results in a ubiquitous focal thickening of the intima, a developmental process that may predispose to later atheroma [13]. In childhood, fatty dots or streaks known as foam cells appear in the subendothelium of the intima, caused by the accumulation of lipid-containing monocytes. The death of these cells results in extravasation of lipid, formation of an extracellular lipid core and stimulation of smooth muscle cell migration and proliferation. This smooth muscle cell proliferation is accompanied by synthesis of structural components of the extracellular matrix, which encapsulate the lipid pool to form the fibrous cap of the more advanced plaque [14]. The proliferation and intimal migration of smooth muscle cells, with concomitant synthesis of elastin, collagen and glycosaminoglycans, may be a reparative response to vascular damage induced by the toxic effects of oxidized low-density lipoproteins and could be integral to the maintenance of plaque stability.

Plaque stability

Full development of an atheromatous plaque may take years, whereas plaque rupture, which can result in coronary thrombosis, myocardial ischaemia and infarction, usually happens suddenly. It seems likely, therefore, that the factors which convert a stable plaque to an unstable one are different from those that influence long-term plaque formation (Fig. 1.3).

It is suggested that the rupture of an advanced atherosclerotic plaque results from the combined effects of intrinsic and extrinsic weakening of the fibrous cap [15]. The former relates to changes in the composition of the plaque itself and the latter to the shear stress of arterial pulsation, especially when systemic pressure is high, which probably precipitates rupture of 'fragile plaques' [16].

Ruptured plaques have increased concentrations of lipid and monocytes and reduced collagen and vascular smooth muscle content [17]. Studies show evidence for a relationship between the size of the subintimal pool of lipid and the number of monocytes and increased tendency to plaque rupture [18,19]. Others indicate that vascular smooth muscle proliferation and collagen formation are linked to vascular repair and plaque stabilization [17,20].

Thus, we might conjecture that plaque stability will be enhanced by processes or agents that aid smooth muscle cell proliferation and synthesis and reduce shear stress, preserving the integrity of the fibrous cap, and reduced by those that increase deposition of lipid and accumulation of monocytes in the intima.

Factors influencing plaque formation and stability	
Plaque formation	**Plaque stability**
• Vascular smooth muscle proliferation	• Intrinsic structural changes to the fibrous cap
• Monocyte and lipid accumulation	• Increased arterial pressure, flow turbulence and vascular deformation
• Cell death	• Increased lipid and monocyte concentration
• Synthesis of extracellular matrix proteins to form the fibrous cap	• Decreased vascular smooth muscle content and collagen content

Fig. 1.3. Factors influencing plaque formation and rupture.

In this context the effects of angiotensin-converting enzyme (ACE) and kininase II inhibition may be of importance. Cell culture studies show that ACE/kininase II inhibition increases the formation of vascular smooth muscle collagen, possibly via modulation of the smooth muscle cell phenotype from a predominantly contractile cell to one that secretes collagen. [21]. Furthermore, the reparative growth rate of endothelial cells may be enhanced by ACE/kininase II inhibition via an increase in the rate of cell migration [22]. In culture, angiotensin II stimulates vascular smooth muscle hypertrophy, possibly via increased expression of the proto-oncogenes c-*myc* and c-*fos* and the A chain of platelet-derived growth factor (PDGF) [23]. There is little evidence, though, *in vitro* for a role for angiotensin II in promoting the proliferation of smooth muscle cells. Should any of these effects occur *in vivo*, they might be expected to alter the stability of atherosclerotic plaques.

Experimental data from animal studies indicate that ACE inhibition may have specific anti-atherosclerotic effects, preventing the initial formation of atherosclerotic plaques. An early study of cholesterol-fed rabbits showed no benefit from ACE inhibition with captopril on aortic atherosclerosis [24] but a more recent study using Watanabe-heritable-hyperlipidaemic rabbits showed a potent anti-atherosclerotic action of captopril after 9 months of treatment [25]. The greatest reduction in the number of atherosclerotic lesions was seen in the descending thoracic aorta and was accompanied by a reduced cholesterol content of lesions. Also, the arterial lesions that persisted in the treated animals had a reduced monocyte content and increased extracellular matrix content compared with controls. Similar results with captopril have been obtained in cholesterol-fed cynomolgus monkeys, a model closer to human atherosclerosis [26].

Anti-atherosclerotic effects have been observed using ACE inhibitors other than captopril. In a study of adult minipigs fed an atherogenic diet [27], perindopril significantly prevented the development of atherosclerosis in the abdominal aorta, left interventricular coronary artery (LIVCA) and brachiocephalic trunk (BCT) by decreasing the cross-sectional area of lesions as well as the number of lipid-laden cells.

The non-sulphydryl ACE inhibitor enalapril, given to cholesterol-fed rabbits for 3 months at non-hypotensive doses (10 mg/kg per day), significantly reduced the percent plaque areas in the thoracic aortas of treated animals compared with controls (31.1% versus 86.8%,

$P < 0.001$ [28]. Aortic cholesterol content was also reduced (controls 31.4 mg/g tissue versus treated 7.4 mg/g tissue, $P < 0.001$), although enalapril had no significant effect on plasma lipid levels.

The mechanisms that underlie the apparent anti-atherosclerotic effects of ACE inhibition are not yet fully elucidated but a number of candidate mechanisms have been proposed (Fig. 1.4) and are now the subject of further studies. Clinical trials are now being done [29] to assess whether ACE inhibition can significantly reduce atherosclerotic disease and its sequelae in humans.

ACE inhibition and atherosclerosis mechanisms
Blood pressure reduction (cf. β-blockers, Ca^{2+} antagonists)
Reduced arterial permeability and lipoprotein entry
Growth factor inhibition (Ang II, PDGF, a and b FGF, EGF, TGFβ etc.)
Bradykinin accumulation (PGI2, EDRF: growth inhibitors)
Free radical scavenging (sulphydryl group) antioxidant for LDL
Anti-inflammatory effect
Ang II, angiotensin II; PDGF, platelet-derived growth factor; EGF, epidermal growth factor; a and b FGF, acidic and basic fibroblast growth factor; TGFβ, transforming growth factor beta; PGI2, prostaglandin I2; EDRF, endothelium-derived relaxing factor; LDL, low-density lipoprotein

Fig. 1.4. Possible mechanisms to explain observed anti-atherosclerotic effects of ACE inhibition. Published by permission [58].

Genetic factors predisposing to myocardial infarction

Epidemiological studies, most notably the Framingham Heart Study, indicate that family history of coronary heart disease is a major risk factor for myocardial infarction. More recently, Cambien and colleagues [30] reported a deletion polymorphism in intron 16 of the ACE gene (*DD*) that was associated with an increased risk of myocardial infarction (odds ratio 3.2) in a subgroup of the population who had suffered an infarction despite being at low risk on established criteria. Due to the relatively small size of the population studied, the finding awaits independent confirmation.

The reasons behind this observed epidemiological association are not clear. It has been shown that the ACE gene polymorphism is strongly correlated with levels of circulating enzyme, although the correlation may not be translated into differences in the amount of the active peptide angiotensin II because this depends on both formation and breakdown. Subjects with the *DD* genotype had mean ACE concentrations that were double those of *II* subjects whereas those with the *ID* genotype had intermediate levels. This raises the possibility that genetically determined elevations in serum (and possibly tissue) ACE increase the risk of ischaemic heart disease.

It is also unclear why this genetic risk factor, the *ACE/ID* polymorphism, was only identified in the absence but not in the presence of other well-known risk factors for myocardial infarction. Furthermore, the *DD* genotype has also been associated with hypertrophic cardiomyopathy and sudden death in families with hypertrophic cardiomyopathy [31], and with a requirement for cardiac transplantation in patients with ischaemic or idiopathic dilated cardiomyopathy [32].

To date, therefore, the *DD* genotype has been shown to modify clinical outcome in different ways in two completely different clinical disorders: atheroma, a multifactorial disease of large arteries, and hypertrophic myopathy, a specific genetic disease of the cardiac beta-myosin heavy chain. The implications of these findings and the underlying mechanisms have yet to be fully assessed and investigated.

Prognosis of acute myocardial infarction

Mortality from coronary heart disease (CHD) in the USA, Europe and Australia has roughly halved since the 1960s, when deaths from ischaemic heart disease were at a peak [33], although the death rates are still relatively high, with approximately half of those who die from cardiovascular disease dying of CHD.

It is interesting briefly to examine the reasons for the fall in the death rate from CHD seen in the last 30 years. In the early 1960s the attitude towards treatment of acute myocardial infarction was very negative: specialist coronary-care units were few and far between, active treatment regimes were experimental and the concept of risk factors in the development and prognosis of CHD was embryonic.

A series of studies [34–39] from Auckland, New Zealand, between 1966 and 1981 chronicled the survival rates of patients admitted to hospital with an acute myocardial infarction. In 1966–1967, before the opening of a coronary care unit at the hospital, 22% of patients under 70 years old died in hospital and, in over half of these patients, death was due to presumed arrhythmias. At three years after myocardial infarction the death rate was 28%, rising to 42% at 6 years and 68% after 15 years of follow-up. A similar set of studies by the same authors [40,41] following a group of patients admitted to hospital in 1981–1982 gave a 3-year mortality of 14%, even though the infarctions, as assessed by a coronary prognostic index, were more severe than in the 1966–1967 admissions. Norris and colleagues attribute the improvement in survival after myocardial infarction between the mid-1960s and the mid-1980s to the known effect of five major improvements in the secondary prevention of ischaemic heart disease during this time:

(1) routine treatment in a coronary-care unit for patients with a first infarct or a reinfarction (i.e. the availability of electrocardiogram monitoring, close nurse observation and effective use of the defibrillator);

(2) development of coronary surgery;

(3) use of beta blockers as routine therapy after infarction;

(4) better understanding and more prompt treatment of the haemodynamic complications of myocardial infarction.

(5) recognition of cigarette smoking as a reversible risk factor.

Despite the relative success of the approaches outlined earlier, it took the advent of thrombolytic therapy in the late 1980s to make further impact on the early survival chances of those suffering either a first acute myocardial infarction or a re-infarction. The first large randomized trials of intravenous streptokinase [42,43] showed a reduction in mortality rate (mortality risk reduction 18%, $P = 0.0002$, at 21 days after infarction in Gruppo Italiano per lo Studio della Sopravvivenza nell'Infarto Miocardio (GISSI) [42] and 25% reduction in the odds of death at 35 days after infarction in International Studies of Infarct Survival (ISIS)-2 [43]) and a limitation in myocardial damage after infarction in survivors [44]. These results have been born out by later studies of intravenous streptokinase and, more recently, tissue plasminogen activator (tPA) [45–53], all of which show lower early mortality after myocardial infarction with thrombolytic treatment. Because death from myocardial infarction in hospital is only the tip of the iceberg of coronary death in the community, the impact of thrombolysis (and aspirin) cannot account for the extent of the apparent reduction.

Most recently, Stevenson *et al.* [54] have recorded the prognosis and determinants of outcome since the introduction of thrombolysis in patients with acute myocardial infarction admitted to a district general hospital in London, UK. Of the 608 patients included in the study, 14.6% died in hospital. Follow-up data (up to 3 years) were available in 596 patients.

All-cause mortality at 30 days, 1 year and 3 years was 16.0%, 21.7% and 29.4%, respectively. Although 3-year mortality in patients treated with thrombolysis was considerably lower than in those who were not (23.3% compared with 45.7%), the percentage of deaths for all patients was similar to that found by Norris *et al.* in their analysis of their 1966–1967 intake of patients with an acute myocardial infarction at 29.4%. Obviously the patients receiving or not receiving thrombolysis are not directly comparable because randomization was not part of this observational study.

Further analysis of their data led Stevenson *et al.* to conclude that although thrombolysis has had an impact on early death after myocardial infarction (the overall 30-day mortality in their study was lower than that reported before thrombolysis was introduced), the chances of long-term survival are not much greater than they were before thrombolysis was introduced in the late 1980s.

There are problems in directly comparing long-term data from present-day and earlier prognostic studies because many of the earlier data relate to patients surviving to hospital discharge, and there are problems with patient comparability. Also, there is only limited information on long-term prognosis after myocardial infarction; de Vreede *et al.* [55], in their meta-analysis of pre-thrombolysis studies of prognosis after myocardial infarction, were able to identify 12 reports since 1960 that looked at long-term survival. From these, they found no evidence that long-term prognosis had improved between 1960 and 1970, the average 5-year mortality data remaining constant.

Subgroup analysis in the study from Stevenson *et al.* [54] reveal some interesting prognostic data. The variables associated with outcome were similar to those reported before thrombolysis was introduced, except for thrombolysis itself and aspirin (Fig. 1.5). Of these variables, the most important was left ventricular failure defined on clinical criteria, a factor that is now well established as a powerful predictor of outcome after myocardial infarction (Fig. 1.6). Advanced age was a second important factor. Other factors, known to affect

---

Factors affecting outcome after MI at 6 months

- Left ventricular failure

- Not receiving thrombolysis

- Not receiving aspirin

- Left bundle branch block

- Age over 60 years

Fig. 1.5. Multivariate analysis of data from [54] shows the factors listed here to be the most important determinants of early (six-month) mortality after myocardial infarction (MI).

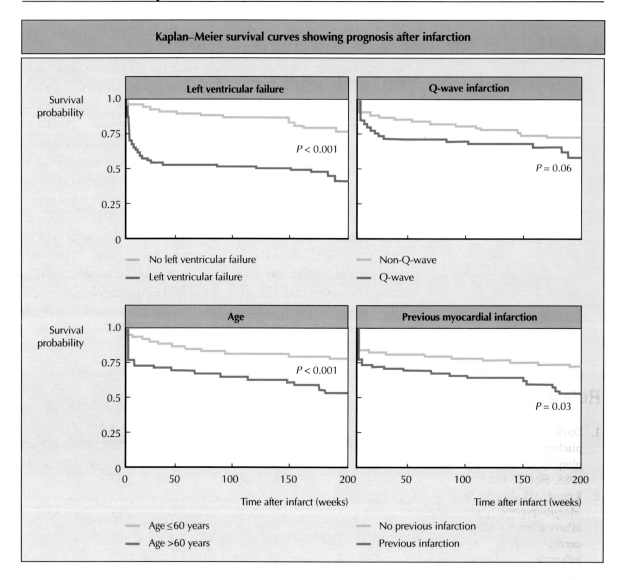

Fig. 1.6. Kaplan–Meier survival curves showing the effects of left ventricular failure, age, Q-wave infarction and previous history of myocardial infarction on prognosis after infarction. The presence of left ventricular failure after infarction was the factor most strongly associated with a worse prognosis. Published by permission [54].

outcome, such as continued remodelling and dilatation of the left ventricle, were not included in the analysis. Curiously, non-smokers fared worse in terms of risk of early death than smokers, although this finding is consistent with earlier data from Thrombolysis in Myocardial Infarction (TIMI)-II [46]. The risk of re-infarction, however, was higher in patients who continued to smoke after the first infarction than in those who stopped smoking.

It is clear from the data presented here that, despite advances in coronary care and the advent of beta blockers, thrombolysis and aspirin, there is room for improvement in the available treatments to increase long-term survival after myocardial infarction, particularly in that subgroup of patients who exhibit clinical heart failure with the associated high risk of fatal and non-fatal ischaemic, arrhythmic and haemodynamic events. Strategies to identify these patients correctly need to be developed but some progress has been made towards additional treatment benefit with the introduction of ACE inhibition after myocardial infarction as a viable treatment option.

This book will review the theoretical evidence for the perceived benefits of ACE inhibition after myocardial infarction (after the initial disappointments of the Cooperative North Scandinavian Enalapril Survival Study (CONSENSUS)-II) and the hard evidence from large-scale clinical trials, and will discuss the clinical implications of the findings from these trials.

References

1. Davies MJ, Woolf N, Rowles PM, Pepper J: **Morphology of the endothelium over atherosclerotic plaques in human coronary arteries.** *Br Heart J* 1988, **60**:459–464.

2. Kragel AH, Reddy SG, Witted JT, Roberts WC: **Morphometric analysis of the composition of atherosclerotic plaques in the four major epicardial coronary arteries in acute myocardial infarction and in sudden coronary death.** *Circulation* 1989, **80**:1747–1756.

3. Davies M, Woolf N, Robertson W: **Pathology of acute myocardial infarction with particular reference to occlusive coronary thrombi.** *Br Heart J* 1976, **38**:659–664.

4. Chapman I: **The cause–effect relationship between recent coronary artery occlusion and acute myocardial infarction.** *Am Heart J* 1974, **87**:267–271.

5. DeWood M, Spores J, Notske R, *et al.*: **Prevalence of total coronary occlusion during the early hours of transmural myocardial infarction.** *N Engl J Med* 1980, **303**:897–902.

6. Stadius M, Maynard C, Fritz J: **Coronary anatomy amd left ventricular function in the first 12 hours of acute myocardial infarction: the Western Washington randomised intracoronary strepto-** kinase trial. *Circulation* 1985, **72**:292–301.

7. Forrester J, Litvak F, Grundfest W, *et al.*: **A perspective of coronary artery disease seen through the arteries of a living man.** *Circulation* 1985, **75**:505–513.

8. Sherman C, Litvak F, Grundfest W: **Coronary angioscopy in patients with unstable pectoris.** *N Engl J Med* 1986, **315**:913–919.

9. Deupree R, Fields R, McMahon C, Strong J: **Atherosclerotic lesions and coronary heart disease. Key relationships in necroscopied cases.** *Lab Invest* 1973, **28**:252–262.

10. Glagov S, Weisenberd E, Zarins C, Stankunvicius R, Kollettis G: **Compensatory enlargement of human atherosclerotic arteries.** *N Engl J Med* 1987, **316**:1317–1375.

11. Ambrose JA, Winters SL, Arora RR, *et al.*: **Angiographic evolution of coronary artery morphology in unstable angina.** *J Am Coll Cardiol* 1986, **7**:472–478.

12. Ambrose JA, Tannenbaum MA, Alexopoulos D, *et al.*: **Angiographic progression of coronary artery disease and the development of myocardial infarction.** *J Am Coll Cardiol* 1988, **12**:56–62.

13. Stary H: **Evolution and progression of**

atherosclerotic lesions in coronary arteries of young children and young adults. *Arteriosclerosis* 1989, **9**:1–19.

14. Mosse PRL, Campbell GR, Wang ZL, Campbell JH: **Smooth muscle phenotypic expression in carotid arteries. I. Comparisons of cells from diffuse intimal thickenings adjacent to atheromatous plaques with those of the media.** *Lab Invest* 1985, **53**:556–562.

15. Fuster V, Stein B, Ambrose J, Badimon L, Badimon JJ, Chesebro JH: **Atherosclerotic plaque rupture and thrombosis: evolving concepts.** *Circulation* 1990, **82** (suppl II):II47–II59.

16. Richardson PD, Davies MJ, Born GVR: **Influence of plaque configuration and stress distribution on fissuring of coronary atherosclerotic plaques.** *Lancet* 1989, **3**:941–944.

17. Davies MJ, Woolf N: **Atherosclerosis: what is it and why does it occur?** *Br Heart J* 1993, **69** (suppl):S1–S11.

18. Brown BG, Zhao XQ, Sacco DE, Albers JJ: **Lipid lowering and plaque regression. New insights into prevention of plaque disruption and clinical events in coronary disease.** *Circulation* 1993, **87**:1781–1790.

19. Lendon C, Davies MJ, Born GVR, Richardson P: **Atherosclerotic plaque caps are locally weakened when macrophage density is increased.** *Atherosclerosis* 1991, **87**:87–90.

20. Badimon JJ, Fuster V, Chesebro JH, Badimon L: **Coronary atherosclerosis. A multifactorial disease.** *Circulation* 1993, **87** (suppl II):II3–II16.

21. Campbell JH, Fennessy P, Campbell GR: **Effect of perindopril on the development of atherosclerosis in the cholesterol-fed rabbit.** *Clin Exp Pharmacol Physiol* 1992, **19**:13–17.

22. Bell L, Madri JA: **Influence of the angiotensin system on endothelial and smooth muscle cell migration.** *Am J Pathol* 1990, **137**:7–12.

23. Naftilan AJ, Pratt RE, Dzau VJ: **Angiotensin II induction of c-Fos, c-Myc platelet-derived growth factor (PDGF) [abstract].** *Clin Res* 1988, **36**:303A.

24. Overturf Ml, Syberg HD, Smith SA: **Captopril-induced hyper-renaemia in cholesterol fed rabbits.** *Res Commun Chem Pathol Pharmacol* 1985, **47**:229–253.

25. Chobanian AV, Haudenschild CC, Nickerson C, Drago R: **Antiatherogenic effect of captopril in the Watanabe heritable hyperlipidaemic rabbit.** *Hypertension* 1990, 15:327–331.

26. Aberg G, Ferrer P: **Effects of captopril on atherosclerosis in cynomolgus monkeys.** *J Cardiovasc Pharmacol* 1990, **15** (suppl 5):S65–S72.

27. Charpiot P, Rolland PH, Friggi A, *et al.*: **ACE inhibition with perindopril and atherogenesis-induced structural and functional changes in minipig arteries.** *Arterioscler Thromb* 1993, **13**:1125–1138.

28. Schuh JR, Blehm DJ, Frierdich GE, McMahon EG, Blaine EH: **Differential effects of renin-angiotensin system blockade on atherogenesis in cholesterol-fed rabbits.** *J Clin Invest* 1993, **91**: 1453–1458.

29. Texter M, Lees RS, Pitt B, Dinsmore RE, Uprichard AC: **The QUinapril Ischaemic Event Trial (QUIET) design and methods: evaluation of chronic ACE inhibitor theory after coronary artery intervention.** *Cardiovasc Drugs Ther* 1993, **7**:273–282.

30. Cambien F, Poirier O, Lecerf L, *et al.*: **Deletion polymorphism in the gene for angiotensin-converting enzyme is a potent risk factor for myocardial infarction.** *Nature* 1992, **359**: 641–644.

31. Marain AJ, Yu Q-T, Workamn R, Greve G, Roberts R: **Angiotensin converting enzyme polymorphism in hypertrophic cardiomyopathy and sudden cardiac death.** *Lancet* 1993, **342**:1085–1086.

32. Raynolds MV, Bristow MR, Bush EW, *et al.*: **Angiotensin-converting enzyme DD genotype in patients with ischaemic or idiopathic dilated cardiomyopathy.** *Lancet* 1993, **342**:1073–1076.

33. Thom TJ: **International mortality from heart disease: rates and trends.** *Int J Epidemiol* 1989, **18** (suppl 1):S20–S28.

34. Norris RM, Bensley KE, Caughey DE, Scott PJ: **Hospital mortality in acute myocardial infarction.** *BMJ* 1968, **3**:143–146.

35. Norris RM, Brandt PWT, Caughey DE, *et al.*: **A new coronary prognostic index.** *Lancet* 1969, **i**:274–278.

36. Norris RM, Brandt PWT, Lee AJ: **Mortality in a coronary-care unit analyzed by a new coronary prognostic index.** *Lancet* 1969, **i**:278–281.

37. Norris RM, Caughey DE, Deeming LW, *et al*: **Coronary prognostic index for predicting survival after recovery from acute myocardial infarction.** *Lancet* 1970, **i**:485–488

38. Norris RM, Caughey DE, Mercer CJ, Scott PJ: **Prognosis after myocardial infarction. Six year follow-up.** *Br Heart J* 1974, **36**:786–790.

39. Merrilees MA, Scott PJ, Norris RM: **Prognosis after myocardial infarction: results of 15-year follow up.** *BMJ* 1984, **288**:355–359.

40. Stewart AW, Fraser J, Norris RM, Beaglehole R: **Changes in severity of myocardial infarction and 3 year survival rates after myocardial infarction in Auckland 1966–67 and 1981–82.** *BMJ* 1988, **297**:517–519.

41. Stewart AW, Fraser J, Norris RM, Beaglehole R, **Improved prognosis after myocardial infarction 1981 vs 1966.** *Circulation* 1988, **78** (suppl II):468.

42. GISSI Trial Group: **Effectiveness of intravenous thrombolytic treatment in acute myocardial infarction.** *Lancet* 1986, **i**:397–401.

43. ISIS-2 (Second International Study of Infarct Survival) Collaborative Group: **Randomised trial of intravenous streptokinase, oral aspirin, both or neither among 17 187 cases of suspected myocardial infarction. ISIS 2.** *Lancet* 1988, **ii**:349–359.

44. White HD, Norris RM, Brown MA, *et al.*: **Effect of intravenous streptokinase on left ventricular function and early survival after acute myocardial infarction.** *N Engl J Med* 1987, **317**:850–855.

45. Chesebro JH, Knutterud G, Roberts R, *et al.*: **Thrombolysis in myo-cardial infarction (TIMI) trial. Phase 1: A comparison between intravenous tissue plasminogen activator and intravenous streptokinase.** *Circulation* 1987, **76**: 142–154.

46. The TIMI Study Group: **Comparison of invasive and conservative strategies after treatment with intravenous tissue plasminogen activator in acute myocardial infarction. Results of the thrombolysis in myocardial infarction (TIMI) phase II trial.** *N Engl J Med* 1989, **320**:618–627.

47. Wilcox RG: **Thrombolysis with tissue plasminogen activator in suspected acute myocardial infarction. The ASSET Study.** *Chest* 1989, **95** (suppl):2705–2755.

48. Topol EJ, Califf RM, George BS, *et al.*: **A randomized trial of immediate versus delayed elective angioplasty after intravenous tissue plasminogen activator in acute myocardial infarction.** *N Engl J Med* 1987: **317**:581–588.

49. Topol EJ, Califf RM, George BS, *et al.*: **Coronary arterial thrombolysis with combined infusion of recombinant tissue-type plasminogen activator and urokinase in patients with acute myocardial infarction.** *Circulation* 1988, **77**:1100–1107.

50. Topol EJ, George BS, Keriakes DJ, *et al.*: **A randomized controlled trial of intravenous tissue plasminogen activator and intravenous heparin in acute myocardial infarction.** *Circulation* 1989, **79**:281–286.

51. Califf R, Topol EJ, Kereiakes DJ, *et al.*: **Long-term outcome in the thrombolysis and angioplasty in myocardial infarction trial.** *Circulation* 1987, **76** (suppl IV):IV260.

52. Muller DW, Topol EJ, George BS, *et al.*: **Long-term follow-up in the Thrombolysis and Angioplasty in Acute Myocardial Infarction (TAMI) trials. Comparison of trials with thrombolysis alone.** *Circulation* 1898, **80** (suppl II):II520.

53. The ISAM Study Group: **A prospective trial of intravenous strepto-kinase in acute myocardial infarction (ISAM). Mortality, morbidity and infarct size at 21 days.** *N Engl J Med* 1986, **314**:1465–1471.

54. Stevenson R, Ranjadayalan K, Wilkinson P, Roberts R, Timmis AD: **Short and long term prognosis of acute myocardial infarction since introduction of thrombolysis.** *BMJ* 1993, **307**:349–353.

55. de Vreede JJM, Gorgels APM, Verstaten GMP, Vermeer F, Dassen WRM, Wellens HJJ: **Did prognosis after myocardial infarction change during the past 30 years? A meta-analysis.** *J Am Coll Cardiol* 1991, **18**:698–706.

56. Braunwald E (ed.): *Heart Disease: A Textbook of Cardiovascular Medicine.* Philadelphia: WB Saunders Co., 1980.

57. Davies MJ: **The progression of atherosclerosis – role of plaque fissuring and thrombosis.** In *New Horizons in Coronary Heart Disease* edited by Born GVR and Schwartz CJ. London: Current Science, 1993, pp 10a.1–10a.8.

58. Sharpe N: **The effects of ACE inhibitors in the progression of atherosclerosis.** *J Cardiol Pharmacol* 1993, **22** (suppl 9):S9–S12.

13

2

Principles of cardiac remodelling

The heart is an organic muscular pump. As such, it is able to remodel itself according to the prevailing physiological and pathological demands. Important questions about remodelling include the following. By what criteria and towards what objectives does cardiac remodelling proceed? By what mechanisms and through what processes do these remodelling processes occur? For clinicians in particular, two further relevant questions must be answered. How can we identify when the remodelling process deviates from the adaptive to the maladaptive? How should we modify the remodelling process to enhance cardiac function and patient longevity?

Definitions of cardiac remodelling

Before discussing the mechanisms and consequences of cardiac remodelling it is necessary to define the term 'remodelling'.

Cardiac remodelling can be taken to refer to intrinsic alterations in the shape and size of the heart and its microstructure in response to pressure and volume overload – for example, hypertension and outflow-tract stenosis (pressure overload) and valvular regurgitation, arteriovenous malformation or chronic anaemia (volume overload) – as well as non-haemodynamic factors (for example, neurohormonal, growth, ischaemic and necrotic factors).

Remodelling is often generally considered by cardiologists to refer to adverse structural changes in ventricular walls, and therefore as something to be vigorously prevented or reversed in all cases. It should be remembered, however, that remodelling is initially a beneficial adaptive response and a distinction between physiological and pathological remodelling is a helpful one.

Physiological remodelling

Physiological remodelling allows the enhancement or maintenance of the pumping capacity of the heart. When sustained increased circulatory demands are made on the heart, as, for example, in athletic training, cardiac pumping capacity can be increased.

The type, intensity and duration of athletic training affects the way in which the left ventricle remodels. Isotonic endurance exercise (such as running) results in volume-overloaded eccentric hypertrophy of the left ventricle [1] whereas isometric resistance training (such as weight-lifting) results in pressure-overloaded concentric hypertrophy [2] (Fig. 2.1).

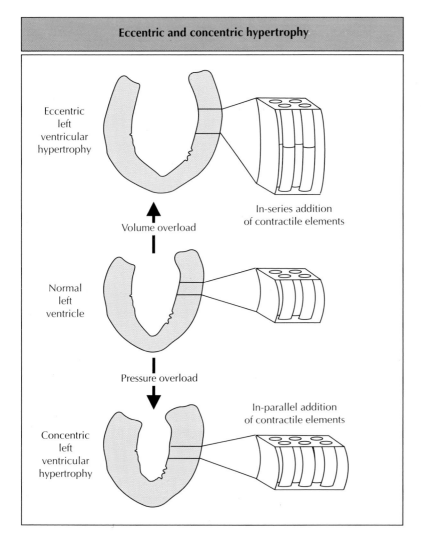

Eccentric and concentric hypertrophy

Eccentric left ventricular hypertrophy

Volume overload

In-series addition of contractile elements

Normal left ventricle

Pressure overload

Concentric left ventricular hypertrophy

In-parallel addition of contractile elements

Fig. 2.1. Concentric left ventricular hypertrophy induced by pressure overload in order to normalize ventricular wall stress while generating greater pressure within the chamber, and eccentric hypertrophy in order to facilitate greater stroke volume output with each sarcomere shortening to the same extent during systole as before hypertrophy.

Eccentric hypertrophy arises because the heart has remodelled itself to ensure that large stroke volumes can be delivered during extreme exertion. Each sarcomere has a maximum shortening distance and so the stroke volume can be increased by increasing the number of in-series sarcomeres.

Concentric hypertrophy occurs because the heart has remodelled itself so that large increases in blood pressure can be generated (mean arterial pressure has been shown to rise to over 160 mmHg during maximal isometric deadlifts, the sort of training that results in concentric hypertrophy [3]). Each myofibril has only a limited capacity to develop tension and so greater wall tension and intraventricular pressure can be generated by increasing the number of in-parallel myofibrils and thus wall thickness.

Exercise that involves both isotonic and isometric components (such as cycling or rowing) results in a combination of concentric and eccentric left ventricular hypertrophy.

When the heart sustains damage that impairs its functional capacity (for example, after myocardial infarction or as a result of valve disease) the ventricular muscle remodels in an attempt to maintain normal circulatory capacity.

Is all left ventricular dilatation necessarily detrimental? In a study of left ventricular volumes during rest and exercise, Crawford and colleagues [4] showed that competitive marathon runners (with a graded bicycle exercise time of 27–33 minutes) had larger left ventricular volumes than non-competitive runners (with a bicycle exercise time of 12–33 minutes), at rest and throughout all stages of exercise. Indeed, the left ventricular end-diastolic volume correlated well with maximum exercise duration (r = 0.80). An earlier study also showed that professional racing cyclists had total heart volumes over 35% greater than those of untrained men [5]. These athletes would no doubt be aggrieved if their enlarged hearts were reduced to the size of those of sedentary subjects!

It appears that ventricular dilatation and hypertrophy can be either physiological and compensatory or pathological (Fig. 2.2). Physiological ventricular remodelling (either dilatation or hypertrophy) is adaptive, compensatory, beneficial and appropriate, whereas pathological remodelling is detrimental and adverse. It is the latter that requires treatment and prevention, not the former.

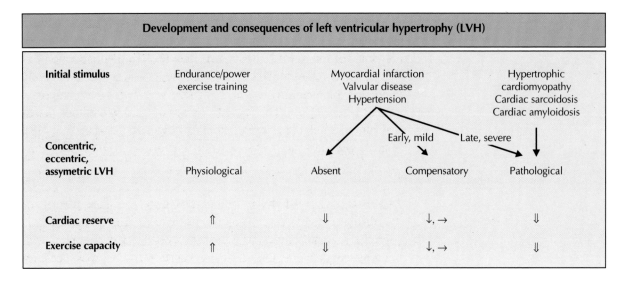

Fig. 2.2. Different modes of development and consequences of left ventricular hypertrophy.

Pathological remodelling

Pathological remodelling by definition results in deterioration in cardiac function. It can be divided into two parts:

- remodelling resulting from alterations in cardiac structure as a result of primary heart disease
- remodelling resulting from secondary physiological processes which have become excessive, counterproductive and therefore detrimental.

Myocardial infarction, infarct extension and expansion represent pathological remodelling. The loss of myocardial mass results in compensatory dilatation of the left ventricle to maintain stroke volume (physiological remodelling). However, if this dilatation becomes excessive (pathological remodelling), complications such as higher myocardial tension–development energy cost, functional mitral regurgitation and tachyarrythmias develop.

Assessment of ventricular remodelling

Modern cardiac imaging techniques allow relatively easy measurement and identification of alterations in the three-dimensional structure of the heart. Echocardiography is the most accessible, but computed tomography and magnetic resonance imaging are more accurate.

Given that it is not always possible at present to distinguish between physiological and pathological hypertrophy after a morphological diagnosis of left ventricular hypertrophy (LVH), the distinction has to be made by assessing the overall function of the heart. A relatively good way of assessing cardiac function is to measure changes in cardiac reserve [6,7]. This has advantages over other methods in that it accounts for changes in pressure and flow-generating capacity [8], systolic and diastolic dysfunction, at-rest function and function during maximal stress.

As already described, myocyte alignment depends on the integrity of the fibrillar network of collagen in the myocardium. If the matrix is degraded or insufficiently strong to preserve myocyte alignment, wall thinning can occur despite myocyte hypertrophy. On gross measurement of wall thickness, it might be concluded that no hypertrophy or remodelling had occurred when in fact the opposite may be true, as in idiopathic dilated cardiomyopathy.

To date there are no imaging techniques that provide reliable information on myocardial ultrastructure, although the possibilities of ultrasound imaging have been explored [9,10]. Information on the impact of ventricular remodelling on the ultrastructure can be assessed only by histological examination of endomyocardial biopsy samples, hearts from cadavers, transplant recipients and animal studies.

Mechanisms of cardiac remodelling

Role of the myocytes, vessels and interstitium

The myocardium can be thought of as consisting of three compartments:

- the myocytes
- the vessels
- the interstitium.

The myocytes are the only mechanically active cell type producing force and shortening by contraction. The vessels and interstitium provide the necessary infrastructure for the myocytes to function optimally.

The interstitium consists of mast cells, macrophages and fibroblasts and the cellular products of the latter, collagen and elastin. The network of collagen and elastin fibres provides the myocardium with its structural integrity, contributing to synchronous contraction of the myofibrils by linking them together and preventing overstretching [11,12]

Interstitial fibroblasts secrete predominantly thick fibres of type I collagen and thin fibres of type III and type IV collagen, which are organized into three distinct layers:

- Endomysial collagen, which surrounds individual myocytes. Lateral connections (struts) of endomysial collagen link adjacent myocytes, and are believed to contribute to the synchronized contraction of myocytes.
- Perimysial collagen, which surrounds groups of myocytes, creating myofibrils. Lateral strands of perimysial collagen (strands) connect adjacent myofibrils.
- Epimysial collagen, which is the outermost layer and forms a complex network within the subendocardium. It is believed to prevent excessive stretching of the myocardium.

The greater the force of contraction of the ventricle, the stronger the collagen strands and struts need to be to prevent slippage and to transmit the tension from one layer to the next, eventually generating high pressure in the ventricular cavity. Because collagen has a very high tensile strength (greater than that of steel [13]), relatively little amounts are required to fulfil its cytoskeletal role.

Myocardial hypertrophy is influenced by a number of factors (Fig. 2.3). Mechanical or haemodynamic factors are known to have a direct trophic effect on the myocytes [14–16], although the exact mechanism of signal transduction is not known (see pp. 24–25). From the perspective of engineering design one can postulate a direct relationship between arterial pressure (x axis) and hypertrophy (y axis; see Fig. 2.4). The ideal slope for a human heart is not known but the existence of an optimum slope is probable. It is reasonable to postulate that any hypertrophic change along this optimum line is physiological. Deviations from the slope imply some contribution from pathological processes. Any therapeutic intervention should aim to revert the slope towards the ideal.

Endocrine and paracrine factors, such as the catecholamines, angiotensins and endothelins, are known to induce ventricular hypertrophy via direct trophic effects and indirect vasoconstrictor effects. They are also known to stimulate fibroblast proliferation and increased collagen synthesis (see pp. 24–25).

Factors influencing myocardial hypertrophy
• Mechanical
• Endocrine
• Growth
• Genetic

Fig. 2.3. Factors influencing myocardial hypertrophy.

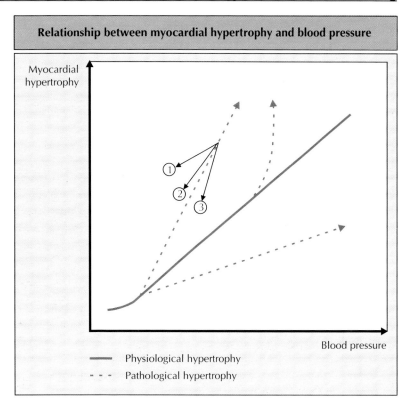

Relationship between myocardial hypertrophy and blood pressure

Fig. 2.4. A schematic representation of the relationship between myocardial hypertrophy and blood pressure. For a given ventricle, there is an optimum slope which reflects physiological hypertrophy as an adaptation to elevated pressure (solid line). If the hypertension is protracted and hypertrophy excessive, or if there are extraneous factors which modify this slope, pathological hypertrophy (broken lines) becomes superimposed on the physiological. Therapy (1, 2, 3) should aim to remove or correct the pathological influences and restore towards the physiological relationship. Departure from this is unlikely to be beneficial.

Growth factors such as basic fibroblast growth factor and insulin-like growth factors [17] are also determinants of myocardial hypertrophy, and may be important in pathological hypertrophy.

The importance of collagen in ventricular remodelling has already been alluded to. In the normal myocardium or in physiological hypertrophy, the concentration of collagen is low. It can be postulated, therefore, that a hypertrophied myocardium with significantly altered collagen must have undergone pathological hypertrophy. An increase in collagen concentration can be caused by selective growth or increased activity of the cardiac fibroblasts or decreased collagen degradation. The functional effect of this increased fibrosis is reduced ventricular compliance. Inducing regression of excess fibrosis is likely to be more difficult to achieve than regression of myocyte hypertrophy. Conversely, a reduction of collagen concentration to below normal is also theoretically possible through differential stimulation of myocyte growth and fibroblast growth in favour of the former, or through an increase in collagenase activity [18]. Excess fibrosis can occur as a result of different mechanisms:

- as a response to cardiomyocyte necrosis: reparative or replacement fibrosis
- as a direct response to the stimulation of hormones or growth factors: reactive fibrosis
- as a response to unknown stimuli or autonomous fibroblast activity: idiopathic fibrosis.

Myocyte cell death is probably the greatest stimulus of fibroblast proliferation and collagen deposition in the myocardium. Its potency is several times greater than that from any stimulus for reactive fibrosis. This is true to such an extent that the occurrence of reactive fibrosis can only be established after prior necrosis has been carefully excluded. Replacing necrotic myocytes in the myocardium with collagen is an important way of preserving ventricular integrity. Suppression of replacement fibrosis can be detrimental, as shown by the tendency to left ventricular aneurysm formation after corticosteroid therapy at the time of acute myocardial infarction [19]. In such a case, the aim of treatment should be to lower blood pressure into the normal range. If hypertrophy is reversed without simultaneous lowering of blood pressure, a maladapted heart may result.

Remodelling in pressure and volume overload

Epidemiological studies of hypertension have reported LVH to be a risk factor, independent of blood pressure levels [20]. This finding has been the single most cited reason in support of the aggressive treatment of LVH. Because it can be easily identified, LVH is now assumed to indicate hypertension-induced damage of the heart. Does this mean that clinicians should strive for regression of all LVH irrespective of how well the hypertension is controlled? In other words, are the three major components of remodelling – cardiomyocyte and ventricular hypertrophy, coronary arterial wall thickening and increased collagen concentration – induced by the elevated pressure itself?

Pressure overload on the heart as exemplified by persistent elevated blood pressure induces mechanical signals for cardiac remodelling [14]. Initially, the ventricular remodelling produced by mechanical stimuli is physiological, as seen in the early stages of hypertension. The cardiomyocytes isolated from such hearts show enhanced performance (remodelling of the myocyte 'compartment') [21].

In the chronic phase, pathological remodelling is superimposed on the initial adaptive response. The combination of medial hypertrophy of the coronary artery (remodelling of the vasculature) and an increase in fibre–capillary ratio (remodelling of the interstitium) make the subendocardial regions of the ventricle more susceptible to ischaemic injury. The excessive neurohormonal activation seen in chronic hypertension not only raises blood pressure but also results in pathological change, such as scattered myocyte necrosis and excessive fibrosis [22,23] (see pp. 24–25). Lowering elevated blood pressure into normal ranges will not in itself prevent or reverse these pathological sequelae. Response to pressure overload may be abnormal because of genetic factors. Elevated blood pressure might act as a trigger to a series of pathological responses, possibly involving local growth factors. Myocyte hypertrophy and collagen deposition may be disproportionate to the mechanical stimulus and be accompanied by misalignment of the myofibrils and collagen fibres.

Removal of the elevated pressure may not be enough to bring about complete resolution of these abnormalities; however, interestingly, administration of a low-dose ACE inhibitor can reduce collagen volume fraction in fibrotic hearts of spontaneously hypertensive rats without significantly lowering blood pressure [24,25].

Volume overload is typified by disorders such as thyrotoxicosis and anaemia, in which total cardiac output is increased, and mitral and aortic regurgitation, in which the left ventricle has to expel regurgitated blood as well as the normal forward flow. The resulting hypertrophy is a dilated overworking left ventricle with eccentric hypertrophy.

The early phases of ventricular remodelling due to volume overload are indistinguishable from physiological hypertrophy and the same detrimental processes as for pressure overload come into play when pathological remodelling is superimposed on the early adaptive remodelling as the volume overload persists.

There is a widespread concept in the literature that dilatation of the left ventricle is detrimental, irrespective of the events initiating the dilatation. To test whether this concept is correct, we can perform a thought experiment. Suppose that, following a sizeable myocardial infarction, the heart were enclosed in a moulded steel case. Would such 'protection' render the heart immune from the effects of volume overload and enhance its ability to maintain a requisite circulation, as compared with a heart without such 'protection'? The answer must be no, because the undilated heart would be less able to maintain adequate stroke volumes especially during exercise. It is not therefore the dilatation itself that needs to be dealt with, but rather the factors (for example, cardiac myocyte necrosis and infarction) precipitating adaptive ventricular dilatation.

In cases of valvular regurgitation, the timing of surgery for such patients is often a perplexing question. We can ask ourselves, 'What level of left ventricular dilatation is excessive?' The answer is that demarcation between physiological and pathological dilatation may vary between individuals. In some patients it may be an end-diastolic left ventricular dimension of 60 mm, whereas in others it may be one of 90 mm. Once the left ventricle begins to fail, the risks of operation have already reached significant levels. It is often recommended that ideally these patients should be operated on just before onset of left ventricular failure but currently there is no satisfactory means of detecting the impending transition.

The role of neurohormonal factors in remodelling

Diverse neurohormonal factors influence cardiac structure, including the renin–angiotensin system (RAS), alpha- and beta-adrenergic stimulation and thyroxine. The RAS in particular appears to be intimately involved in the alteration of left ventricular structure in response to different stimuli.

Angiotensin II is well known to have a direct vasoconstrictive effect, increasing ventricular afterload with the consequences for ventricular structure already described (see pp. 21 and 23). It is also known to stimulate myocyte hypertrophy indirectly via its interaction with sympathetic tone [26].

Both circulating and tissue-specific (cardiac) angiotensin II have a direct trophic effect on cardiac myocytes. Cardiac myocytes *in vitro* and *in vivo* have angiotensin II receptors [27,28]. Angiotensin II stimulates DNA and RNA turnover in isolated myocytes and increased protein synthesis is observed within hours of exposure to angiotensin II [29–31]; these effects are probably modulated by protein kinase C, cytosolic calcium and activation of growth-modulating proto-oncogenes [32,33].

As hinted earlier in the chapter, it is thought that angiotensin II stimulates proliferation of cardiac fibroblasts and concomitant collagen synthesis. In experimental models of hypertension, angiotensin II has been shown to contribute to interstitial myocardial collagen accumulation [11,34].

Perhaps the greatest body of evidence for a role for the RAS, and angiotensin II in particular, lies in the number of studies in animals and humans that have demonstrated reversal of LVH and fibrosis by ACE inhibitors, even at doses below those needed to lower blood pressure in the case of non-hypertensive LVH [35–48].

Finally, it has been shown that at high plasma concentrations angiotensin II is toxic to cardiac myocytes, causing necrosis of the cells, a powerful stimulant to fibroblast proliferation and collagen secretion. Early studies showed that injury to the cardiac myocytes occurs in renal ischaemia [49–51].

Infusion of exogenous angiotensin II at high doses resulted in focal myocardial necrosis [52,53]. More recently, it has been shown that even low doses of exogenous angiotensin II cause myocytolysis and fibroblast proliferation within 2 days in rats, before any effect on arterial blood pressure was noted [54].

References

1. MacFarlane N, Northridge DB, Wright AR, Grant S, Dargie HJ: **A comparative study of left ventricular structure and function in elite athletes.** *Br J Sports Med* 1991, **25**:45–48.
2. Longhurst JC, Stebbins CL: **The isometric athlete.** *Cardiol Clin* 1992, **10**:281–294.
3. Sullivan J, Hanson P, Rakho PS, Folts JD: **Continuous measurement of left ventricular performance during and after maximal isometric deadlift exercise.** *Circulation* 1992, **85**:1406–1413.
4. Crawford MH, Petru MA, Rabinowitz C: **Effect of isotonic exercise training on left ventricular volume during upright exercise.** *Circulation* 1985, **72**:1237–1243.
5. Konig K: **Normal values in adults ergometry according to age, sex and training.** In *Proceedings of Meeting of the Working Group of European Society of Cardiology on Physiology, Physiopathology and Electrocardiography of Exercise* edited by Rulli *et al.* Rome, 1980, p. 81.
6. Tan L-B: **Clinical and research implications of new concepts in the assessment of cardiac pumping performance in heart failure.** *Cardiovasc Res* 1987, **21**:615–622.
7. Tan L-B: **Evaluation of cardiac dysfunction, cardiac reserve and inotropic response.** *Postgrad Med J* 1991, **67** (suppl 1):S10–S20.
8. Shroff SG, Motz W: **Left ventricular systolic resistance in rats with hypertension and hypertrophy.** *Am J Physiol* 1989, **257**:H386–H394.
9. Mimbs JW, O'Donnell M, Bauwens D, Miller JW, Sobel BE: **The dependence of ultrasonic attenuation and back scatter on collagen content in dog and rabbit hearts.** *Circ Res* 1980, **47**:49–58.
10. Miller JG, Perez JE, Sobel BE: **Ultrasonic characterization of myocardium.** *Prog Cardiovasc Dis*

1985, **28**:85–110.

11. Weber KT, Brilla CG: **Pathological hypertrophy and cardiac interstitium: fibrosis and renin–angiotensin–aldosterone system.** *Circulation* 1991, **83**:1849–1865.

12. Weber KT, Clark WA, Janicki JS, Shroff SG: **Physiologic versus pathologic hypertrophy and the pressure overload myocardium.** *J Cardiovasc Pharmacol* 1987, **10** (suppl 6):37–49.

13. Burton AC: **Relation and structure to function of the tissue of the wall of vessels.** *Physiol Rev* 1954, **34**:619–642.

14. Cooper G, Kent RL, Mann DL: **Load induction of cardiac hypertrophy.** *J Mol Cell Cardiol* 1989, **21** (suppl 5):11–30.

15. Komuro I, Kaida T, Shibazaki Y, *et al.*: **Stretching cardiac myocytes stimulates protooncogene expression.** *J Biol Chem* 1990, **625**:3595–3598.

16. Mann DL, Kent RL, Parsons B, Cooper G: **Load regulation of the properties of adult feline cardiocytes: growth induction by celluar deformation.** *Circ Res* 1989, **64**: 1079–1090.

17. Long CS, Kariya K, Karns L, Simpson PC: **Tropic factors for cardiac myocytes.** *Hypertension* 1990, **8** (suppl):S219–S224.

18. Weber KT, Brilla CG. **Pathological hypertrophy and cardiac interstitium.** *Circulation* 1991, **83**:1849–1965.

19. Weber KT, Clark WA, Janicki JS, Shroff SG: **Physiologic versus pathologic hypertrophy and the pressure overload myocardium.** *J Cardiovasc Pharmacol* 1987, **10** (suppl 6):37–49.

20. Kannel WB. **Left ventricular hypertrophy as a risk factor in arterial hypertension.** *Eur Heart J* 1992, **13** (suppl D):82–88.

21. Brooksby P, Levi AJ, Jones JV: **Contractile properties of ventricular myocytes isolated from spontaneously hypertensive rats.** *J Hypertens* 1992, **10**:521–527.

22. Benjamin IJ, Jalil JE, Tan LB, Cho K Weber KT, Clark WA: **Isoproterenol-induced myocardial fibrosis in relation to myocyte necrosis.** *Circ Res* 1989, **65**: 657–670.

23. Tan LB, Jalil JE, Pick R, Janicki JS, Weber KT: **Cardiac myocyte necrosis induced by angiotensin II.** *Circ Res* 1991, **69**:1185–1195.

24. Brilla CG, Janicki JS, Weber KT: **Cardioreparative effects of lisinopril in rats with genetic hypertension and left ventricular hypertrophy.** *Circulation* 1991, **83**:1771–1779.

25. Brilla CG, Janicki JS, Weber KT: **Impaired diastolic function and coronary reserve in genetic hypertension. Role of interstitial fibrosis and medial thickening of intramyocardial coronary arteries.** *Circ Res* 1991b, **69**:107–115.

26. Morgan HE, Baker KM: **Cardiac hypertrophy. Mechanical, neural and endocrine dependence.** *Circulation* 1991, **83**:13–25.

27. Rogers TB, Gaa SH, Allen IS: **Identification and characterization of functional angiotensin II receptors on cultured heart myocytes.** *J Pharmacol Exp Ther* 1986, **236**:438–444.

28. Urata H, Healy B, Stewart RW, Bumpus FM, Husain A: **Angiotensin II receptors in normal and failing human hearts.** *J Clin Endocrinol Metab* 1989, **69**:54–66.

29. Khairallah PA, Robertson AL, Davila D: **Effects of angiotensin II on DNA, RNA and protein synthesis.** In *Hypertension 1972* edited by Genest J, Koiw E. New York: Springer Verlag, 1972, pp 212–218.

30. Aceto JF, Baker KM: **[Sar-1]angiotensin II receptor mediated stimulation of protein synthesis in chick heart cells.** *Am J Physiol* 1990, **258**:H806–H813.

31. Baker KM, Aceto JF: **Angiotensin II stimulation of protein synthesis and cell growth in chick heart cells.** *Am J Physiol* 1990, **259**: H610–618.

32. Hoh E, Komuro I, Kurabayashi M, Katoh Y, Shibazaki Y, Yazaki Y: **The molecular mechanism of angiotenin II-induced c-*fos* gene expression on rat cardiomyocytes [abstract].** *Circulation* 1990, **82** (suppl III):351.

33. Izumo S, Nadal-Ginard B, Mahdavi V: **Proto-oncogene induction and reprogramming of cardiac gene expression produced by pressure overload.** *Proc Natl Acad Sci U S A* 1988, **85**:339–343.

34. Brilla CG, Pick R, Tan LB, Janicki JS, Weber KT: **Remodeling of the rat right and left ventricles in experimental hypertension.** *Circ Res* 1990, **67**: 1355–1364.

35. Fouad FM, Tarazi RC, Bravo EL: **Cardiac and haemodynamic effects of enalapril.** *J Hypertension* 1983, **1** (suppl 1):135–142.

36. Dunn FG, Oigman W, Ventura HO, Messerli FH, Kobrin I, Frohlich ED: **Enalapril improves systemic and renal hemodynamics and allows regression of left ventricular mass in essential hypertension.** *Am J Cardiol* 1984, **53**:105–108.

37. Nakashima Y, Fouad FM, Tarazi RC: **Regression of left ventricular hypertrophy from systemic hy-**

pertension by enalapril. *Am J Cardiol* 1984, **53**:1044–1049.

38. Ventura HO, Frohlich ED, Messerli FH, Kobrin I, Kardon MB: **Cardiovascular effects and regional blood flow distribution associated with angiotensin converting enzyme inhibition (captopril) in essential hypertension.** *Am J Cardiol* 1985, **55**:1023–1026.

39. Sheiban I, Arcaro G, Govi G, Accardi R, Zenorini C, Lechi A: **Regression of cardiac hypertrophy after antihypertensive therapy with nifedipine and captopril.** *J Cardiovasc Pharm* 1987, **10** (suppl 10):S187–S191.

40. Muiesan ML, Agabiti-Rosei E, Romanelli G, Castellano M, Bescht M, Muiesan G: **Beneficial effects of one year's treatment with captopril on left ventricular anatomy and function in hypertensive patients with left ventricular hypertrophy.** *Am J Med* 1988, **84** (suppl 3A):129–132.

41. Trimarco B, De Luca N, Ricciardelli B, *et al.*: **Cardiac function in systemic hypertension before and after reversal of left ventricular hypertrophy.** *Am J Cardiol* 1988, **62**:745–750.

42. Grandi AM, Venco A, Barzizza F, Casadet B, Marches E, Finardi G: **Effect of enalapril on left ventricular mass and performance in essential hypertension.** *Am J Cardiol* 1989, **63**:1093–1097.

43. Sanchez RA, Trabailli CA, Marco EJ, Cianciulli T, Giannone CA, Ramirez AJ: **Long-term evaluation of cilazapril in severe hypertension. Assessment of left ventricular and renal function.** *Am J Med* 1989, **87** (suppl 6B):56–60S.

44. Julien J, Durloux M-A, Prasquer R, *et al.*: **Effects of captopril and minoxidil on left ventricular hypertrophy in resistant hypertensive patients. A 6 month double-blind comparison.** *J Am Coll Cardiol* 1990, **16**:137–142.

45. Schneeweiss A, Rosenthal J, Marmor A: **Comparative evaluation of the acute and chronic effects of cilazapril and hydrochlorothiazide on diastolic cardiac function in hypertensive patients.** *J Human Hypertens* 1990, **4**:35–39.

46. Angermann CE, Spes CH, Willems S, Dominiak P, Kemkes BM., Theisen K: **Regression of left ventricular hypertrophy in hypertensive heart transplant recipients treated with enalapril, furosemide and verapamil.** *Circulation* 1991, **84**:583–593.

47. Grandi AM, Venco A, Barzizza E, *et al.*: **Double-blind comparison of perindopril and captopril in hypertension.** *Am J Hypertens* 1991, **4**:516–520.

48. Schieffer B, Wriger A, Meybrunn M, *et al.*: **Comparative effects of chronic angiotensin-converting enzyme inhibiton and angiotensin II type 1 receptor blockade on cardiac remodelling after myocardial infarction in the rat.** *Circulation* 1994, **89**:2273–2282.

49. Winternitz MC, Mylan, E, Watres LL, Katzenstein R: **Studies on the relation of the kidney to cardiovascular disease.** *Yale J Biol Med* 1940, **12**:623–674.

50. Muirhead EE: **Renal tissue and extracts versus cardiovascular injury.** *Arch Pathol* 1963, **76**:613–619.

51. Bahn RD, Giacomelli F, Wiener J: **Ultrastructure of coronary arteries and myocardium in experimental hypertension.** *Exp Mol Pathol* 1978, **29**:66–81.

52. Gavras H, Brown JJ, Lever AF, MacAdam RF, Robertson JIS: **Acute renal failure, tubular necrosis and myocardial infarction induced in the rabbit by intravenous angiotensin II.** *Lancet* 1971, **ii**:19–22.

53. Gavras H, Kremer D, Brown JJ, *et al.*: **Angiotensin and norepinephrine-induced myocardial lesions: experimental and clinical studies in man.** *Am Heart J* 1975, **89**:321–332.

54. Tan L-B, Jalil JE, Pick R, Janicki JS, Weber KT: **Cardiac myocyte necrosis induced by angiotensin II.** *Circ Res* 1991, **69**:1185–1195.

3

Cardiac remodelling after myocardial infarction: animal and human data

Infarction of the myocardium secondary to coronary artery occlusion is the most common affliction affecting the heart in western society. The infarcted myocardium undergoes conformational changes (thinning and expansion) which, together with the loss of the heart's contribution to the pumping action of the entire ventricle, increases the mechanical loading and triggers complex biological processes. This leads to cardiac remodelling; the larger the infarction, the greater this remodelling. The remodelling processes produce structural, ultrastructural and functional changes, some of which are physiological and compensate for the loss of myocardium and some of which are pathological and lead to detrimental deterioration of function.

Ventricular enlargement after myocardial infarction

The damage to the heart after an acute myocardial infarction, as manifested by the loss of a significant amount of viable myocardium, leads to immediate alterations in wall stress and ventricular topography in both the infarcted region and the remaining viable myocardium, a process of ventricular remodelling. This pattern of post-infarct ventricular remodelling is one of chamber enlargement and distortion of ventricular shape (Fig. 3.1).

The strong association between ventricular enlargement and reduced survival after myocardial infarction has generated interest in the factors associated with ventricular enlargement and the potential treatment strategies to modify the process.

Ventricular enlargement after myocardial infarction is influenced by three closely related factors:

- the degree of loss of myocardium (dependent on infarct size and type of infarct) and infarct expansion

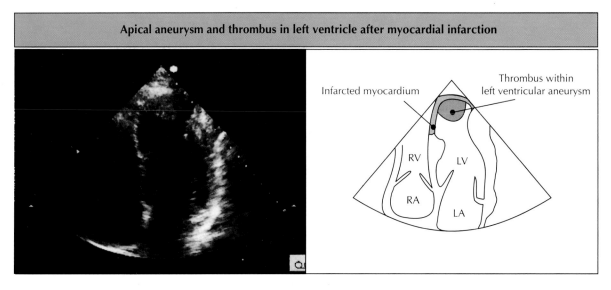

Apical aneurysm and thrombus in left ventricle after myocardial infarction

Fig. 3.1. Echocardiogram of a dilated left ventricle after a large antero-apical myocardial infarction resulting in an apical aneurysm with a thrombus.

- scar formation
- ventricular wall stress.

Degree of myocardial loss and infarct expansion

Myocardial infarction involves necrosis of a region of the myocardium which usually progresses to an inflammatory response and eventual replacement of the contractile myocardium by fibrous tissue. The initial change results in thinning of the infarcted region with a concomitant reduction in the number of myocytes. Not only does the infarcted area thin but it also elongates, a process known as infarct expansion [1]. This expansion both enlarges and distorts the shape of the ventricle.

Transmural infarctions are more likely to result in infarct expansion than non-transmural infarcts. This is especially so in those involving the anteroapical region of the left ventricle because of the reduced radius of curvature and wall thickness of this region [1,2]. Infarct expansion is associated with a greater likelihood of both early and late complications, such as death, myocardial rupture, aneurysm formation, cardiogenic shock, and development of cardiac failure [3–6].

Initially, changes in the non-contractile infarcted region are most apparent (as measured on echocardiography) but, later, changes in the non-infarcted region can be detected [4]. The overall process of enlargement therefore involves both the infarcted and the non-infarcted tissue. In the early stages, the infarcted tissue makes the greatest contribution to ventricular enlargement through 'expansion', but the heart may also dilate through the Frank–Starling mechanism to make up for the loss of functional tissue (see Ventricular wall stress). With time the contribution of the non-infarcted tissue becomes the major contributor to ventricular dilatation [7].

Apart from the increase in ventricular circumference that infarct expansion creates, the change in shape of the ventricle, from an ellipsoidal to a more spherical shape occurring after infarction also contributes to the overall enlargement [8].

Scar formation

During the early period of infarct expansion, that is the thinning and elongation of the non-contractile segment of the myocardium, scar healing occurs, characterized by fibroblast proliferation, collagen deposition and connective tissue repair processes connecting disrupted myocytes (Fig. 3.2). This scar healing increases the tensile strength of the infarcted region, providing resistance to further distortion [9,10]. Once healing has occurred, the tensile properties of the fibrous connective scar tissue are such that it is relatively non-distensible and resistant to further distortion [11].

During scar formation, the infarcted region is particularly vulnerable to other factors. Studies in humans and animals examining the effect of anti-inflammatory agents, especially corticosteroids, given after acute infarction have shown that these agents exacerbate the process of infarct expansion, resulting in thinner scars and greater segment elongation [12–15]. It seems that the detrimental effect on scar formation of these agents is the result of a prolonging of the vulnerable healing period before the infarcted region develops a scar with sufficiently high tensile strength to resist further deformation, rather than any direct effect overall on the eventual scar composition itself [16,17]. However, agents which alter fibroblast proliferation, collagen deposition or resorption may be expected to affect the process of scar formation. ACE inhibition has been reported to reduce myocardial fibrosis directly in myocardium of the spontaneously hypertensive rat [18,19]. It is conceivable that this may have some bearing on the early phase of scar formation after acute myocardial infarction.

Ventricular wall stress

Ventricular wall enlargement to restore stroke volume towards normal to compensate for loss of functional myocardium after acute

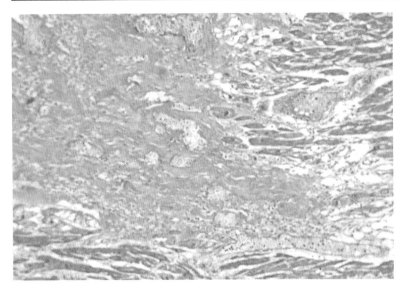

Fig. 3.2. Scar tissue in a 'healing' region of myocardial infarction. After acute myocardial infarction, the necrotic tissue is gradually resorbed, fibroblasts proliferate and collagen is deposited, forming the scar tissue. The process is termed replacement or reparative fibrosis. Collagen is stained blue with Martius scarlet blue staining, while cardiac myocytes stain dark red. Thin-walled blood vessels containing erythrocytes are present in the fibrous tissue. Published by permission [77].

infarction has both immediate and long-term effects. It has particular consequences for, and is influenced by, ventricular wall stress. If the ratio of ventricular mass to ventricular volume is offset towards greater volume per unit mass, ventricular wall stress will be increased at any given pressure level throughout the cardiac cycle. A poorly contracting enlarged ventricle, such as the remodelled post-infarct ventricle, can be viewed as an internally loaded ventricle, as wall stress is constantly increased during the entire cardiac cycle. The impaired ventricle operates from a higher initial radius and exhibits less shortening than the normal ventricle; these factors can lead to an increase in wall stress during ejection rather than the decrease seen in the normal ventricle [20].

Pfeffer and Braunwald have argued that the altered loading state of the remodelled ventricle after infarction may lead to further ventricular enlargement, further increases in wall stress and so on, in a vicious cycle of ventricular dilatation ultimately culminating in heart failure [21] (Fig. 3.3).

In support of this, it is known that modification of haemodynamic factors can have a marked effect on the balance between myocardial oxygen supply and demand during acute infarction. Reduction of ventricular wall stress (and thus oxygen demand) appears to be associated with favourable attenuations in acute infarct expansion as well as the more chronic process of overall ventricular dilatation [22].

It is relevant, however, to ask here whether it is likely that the heart should undergo a remodelling response (which is initially compensa-

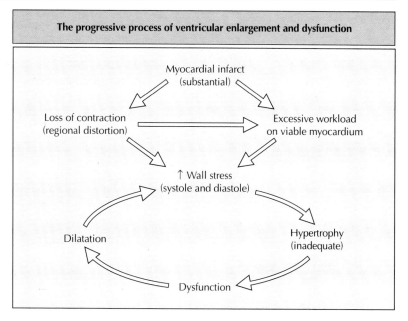

The progressive process of ventricular enlargement and dysfunction

Myocardial infarct (substantial)

Loss of contraction (regional distortion)

Excessive workload on viable myocardium

↑ Wall stress (systole and diastole)

Dilatation

Hypertrophy (inadequate)

Dysfunction

Fig. 3.3. Proposed pathological scheme whereby the loss of substantial myocardium resulting from an acute myocardial infarction can lead to a progressive process of enlargement and dysfunction. In our view this scheme requires modification. Adapted by permission [20].

tory) that culminates in the cardiac pump becoming unstable, as envisaged by Pfeffer and Braunwald? Surely it is more likely that in those instances where the initial insult is of a size to be contained by the compensatory remodelling response, the functional state of the heart will stabilize to a steady-state equilibrium unless that steady state is perturbed by further myocyte necrosis, either as a result of a second infarct or as part of ongoing necrosis in the remaining viable myocardium. For example, once a balloon is inflated and the wall stress in place, the equilibrium is such that further change will only occur if some new event takes place within or outside the walls of the balloon. Unlike the passive property of the balloon wall, the ventricular wall has the capacity to undergo concentric and eccentric hypertrophy, in an attempt to maintain stroke volume and normalize wall stress through active cellular and matrix remodelling. A more likely cause for the progressive ventricular dilatation and dysfunction is further incremental loss of myocardium.

Cardiomyocyte necrosis: a stimulus for cardiac remodelling

Necrosed cardiomyocytes do not regenerate and are replaced by scar tissue. Thus, their loss must be compensated for by reparative processes that seek to produce normal functional capacity from the remaining unimpaired myocardium.

When myocardial necrosis is limited, the main inflammatory response is infiltration of macrophages. The existing microvasculature and reticular framework of myocytes is retained and collagen and proteoglycans are deposited in a process known as reparative or replacement fibrosis. The fibrotic area is smaller than the volume of dead myocytes that it replaces because of the high tensile strength of the collagen fibres. In line with the axiom that nature abhors a vacuum, the surrounding viable myocardium hypertrophies to take up the remaining space, thus minimizing the loss of contractile force caused by the death of a proportion of cardiomyocytes (see Chapter 2).

When myocardial necrosis is more extensive, as in a sizeable myocardial infarct, the initial inflammatory response is quite marked. Key events are myocyte necrosis, inflammation, cellular infiltration and oedema, and breakdown of collagen fibres as a result of activation of collagenases and similar enzymes. The cumulative effect of these responses is to break down the myocardial structure, causing slippage and expansion of the infarcted area.

In addition to scar formation and myocyte hypertrophy, myocyte necrosis is followed by resorption of the dead myocytes, fibroblast proliferation, and formation of new capillaries. In small infarcts when perfusion is adequate and necrosis limited, fibroblast proliferation peaks at days 1-2 after infarct [23]. When arterial occlusion is persistent and the infarct is large, these processes usually start at the periphery because of the inaccessibility of the central zone of large infarcts and the proliferation rate peaks later. Neovascularization secondary to angiogenesis eventually facilitates repair of the central zone.

The role of neurohormonal activation

The sympathetic system and RAS are activated early after an acute myocardial infarction [24-26], but it has also been claimed that significant activation of the RAS occurs later [27]. In most patients, this activation subsides several days after the infarction [27-29] but in patients who have significant left ventricular dysfunction, plasma levels of angiotensin II and noradrenaline remain elevated for a protracted period [26,30]. The concentration of circulating hormones is important but the influence of local catecholamines and angiotensin II in the tissues may be more so.

It is now known that the heart has its own tissue RAS. Renin, angiotensinogen and ACE mRNAs have been identified in mammalian ventricular tissue [31-34]. It has been shown that these mRNAs are translated into proteins and interact to form the peptide, angiotensin II. Lindpaintner and colleagues [35] have shown that ACE inhibition reduces atrial angiotensin II concentrations in nephrectomized rabbits and that angiotensin I is converted to angiotensin II in isolated perfused hearts. The presence of angiotensin II receptors in cardiac tissue is also indicative of a physiologically relevant cardiac RAS [36–43]. Finally, angiotensin II has been shown to be taken up and localized in the nuclei of cardiomyocytes [44], and angiotensin II receptors have been shown to exist in nuclear chromatin [45,46]. Together, these findings suggest that angiotensin II may act indirectly through cell surface receptors and directly on the nucleus to affect fundamental cellular functions.

That overactivation of the tissue RAS is associated with pathophysiological states is demonstrated by several recent pieces of evidence. First, a reduced sodium intake increases renin and angiotensin mRNA expression in the heart [47]. Second, ventricular hypertrophy secondary to pressure overload is associated with a rise in angiotensinogen and ACE mRNA [34,48]. Third, increased cardiac ACE activity is associated with hypertrophy of the left ventricle in rats with aortic banding [49,50] and in heart failure [51]. Finally, cardiac gene expression and ACE activity are increased in rapid pacing-induced heart failure [52]. In addition, we know that angiotensin II may act as a growth factor – both through its cell surface receptors and by binding to nuclear chromatin [44,45], and the c-*mas* oncogene product is similar in structure to the angiotensin receptor [53] – and may have profound effects on the metabolism and proliferation of cardiac fibroblasts, vascular cells and myocyte hypertrophy [54]. It stimulates collagen synthesis and diminishes collagenase activity in cultured rat fibroblasts [55], processes which contribute to pathological ventricular remodelling if allowed to continue unchecked.

Activation of the sympathetic system and RAS after myocardial infarction has positive effects on the myocardium in that it augments pumping performance and maintains adequate circulation. It also stimulates the reparative processes of fibroblast proliferation, collagen synthesis and hypertrophy of viable cardiomyoctes mentioned earlier. Moreover, the sympathetic system and RAS are not independent systems. Angiotensin is known to enhance sympathetic activity, and catecholamines are known to stimulate renin release. In a sense, each system provides positive feedback for the other. However, these positive effects after myocardial infarction can be counteracted by the increased myocardial energy consumption caused by vasoconstriction, hypercontraction and tachycardias, which exacerbate myocardial ischaemia. Catecholamines are also toxic to the cardiac myocytes at high concentrations and excessive and prolonged stimulation may be cumulatively detrimental [56]. There are, however, in-built cellular mechanisms for desensitizing the beta-adrenoreceptors that can diminish this damaging process [57].

Very recently, we have learnt that myocardial angiotensin II levels have been found to be elevated several-fold in the viable myocardium that remains after a large infarction (Hirsch AT, personal communication). These increased concentrations in areas of viable myocardium could induce small scattered areas of myocyte necrosis [23], which could then induce fibrinogenesis, resulting in contracted areas of interstitial and perivascular replacement fibrosis with adjacent myocyte hypertrophy. This continuing loss of myocytes necessitates progressive ventricular dilatation and myocardial hypertrophy to maintain stroke volume.

After acute myocardial infarction, interstitial collagen is increased in the form of replacement fibrosis in non-infarcted myocardium in humans [58,59] and in rats [60,61], suggesting prior myocyte micronecrosis. The appearance of subendocardial fibrosis [60] is similar to that seen after isoprenaline-induced myocyte necrosis [56]: both these findings are in line with the known replacement fibrosis response seen after cardiomyocte necrosis [56,62–64].

Tissue ACE levels are markedly elevated in the infarcted area, but are also significantly increased in non-infarcted regions of viable myocardium [65]. Even at 12 weeks after infarction, increased ACE activity is found in regions that are remote from the infarct site [66]. In rats with a large myocardial infarction, a 6.6-fold rise in angiotensin II receptor mRNA was observed with a 44% increase in the density of angiotensin II receptors in isolated myocytes taken from regions of viable myocardium, accompanied by increased expression of c-*myc* and c-*jun* proto-oncogenes [67]. Expression of angiotensinogen mRNA is increased within one week of experimental myocardial infarction [68].

On the basis of these observations, we can conceive of a sequence of events modulated by overactivation of the sympathetic and renin-angiotensin systems that results in ongoing cardiomyocyte damage with its known consequences on the structure and function of the infarcted heart. This sequence involves scattered replacement fibrosis, compensatory myocyte hypertrophy and progressive dilatation of the left ventricle (Fig. 3.4). Direct proof of this hypothesis is not available but circumstantial evidence supports it.

The role of ACE inhibition in remodelling after myocardial infarction

In experimental models of myocardial infarction in the rat, ACE inhibition has been shown to reduce left ventricular dilatation and ventricular mass [69,70].

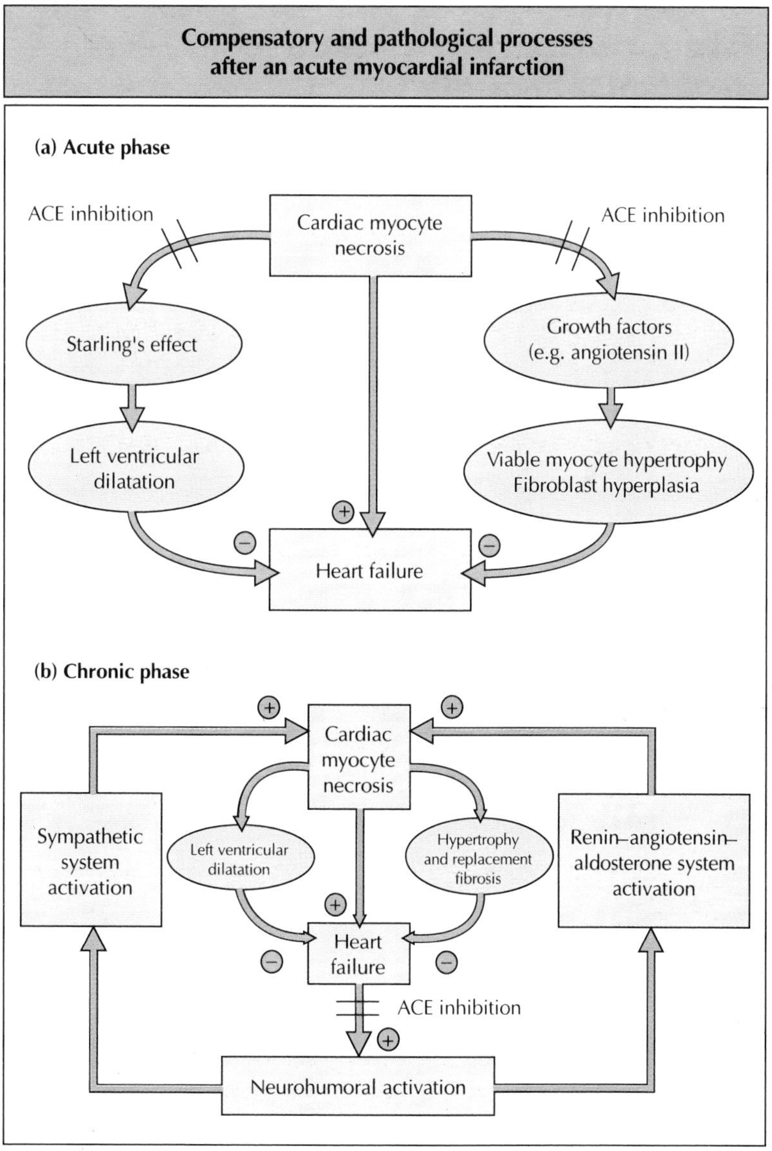

Fig. 3.4. Compensatory and pathological processes occurring after a myocardial infarction. In the acute phase (a), the loss of substantial amounts of cardiac myocytes would lead to heart failure, but this is ameliorated by compensatory ventricular dilatation (haemodynamically induced) and hypertrophy (with associated fibroblast proliferation and collagen deposition through stimulatory growth factors including angiotensin II and noradrenaline). ACE inhibition at this stage diminishes the effects of Starling's mechanism (through vasodilatation) and of neurohumorally mediated myocyte hypertrophy and fibrosis; this may be detrimental. In the chronic phase (b) and in the presence of heart failure, neurohumoral activation becomes persistent and this may lead to on-going cardiomyocyte necrosis which necessitates further ventricular dilatation and replacement fibrosis. ACE inhibition would suppress the on-going necrosis and thereby prevent progressive ventricular dysfunction.

37

Rat models have also shown that ACE inhibitors prevent collagen accumulation [61,69,70]. Furthermore, left ventricular function was improved with decreased left ventricular filling pressures [69,70], normalization of the peak stroke volume index [69] and increased left ventricular ejection fraction [70]. Long-term follow-up of rats subjected to experimental infarction treated with an ACE inhibitor has shown that mortality is reduced, especially in animals with moderate-sized infarctions [71].

Studies in humans of ACE inhibition after myocardial infarction have given similar indications of the benefit of ACE inhibition after myocardial infarction. These are discussed in detail in Chapter 4.

Functional consequences of remodelling after myocardial infarction

The mechanical function of the ventricle is impaired by sizeable myocardial infarction. The haemodynamic consequences of this impairment trigger the remodelling processes, resulting in ventricular dilatation and myocardial hypertrophy. As described in Chapter 2, the stroke volume may be maintained with dilatation and myocardial wall stress may be normalized with hypertrophy. In purely mechanical terms, an equilibrium will be reached if these compensatory remodelling processes were truly compensatory, such that the functional capacity of the ventricle will revert towards or to the pre-infarction state. Any interference of the adaptive processes (for example, by limiting dilatation or hypertrophy) would be detrimental. Furthermore, dilatation or hypertrophy beyond the equilibrium state must indicate maladaptive development.

Gaudron and colleagues studies left ventricular function over 3 years of remodelling after myocardial infarction using single photon emission computed tomography (SPECT) and exercise haemodynamics [72]. In 20% of patients with the worst ventricular function, progressive left ventricular dilatation was noted (Fig. 3.5). Haemodynamic studies showed that, at 4 weeks and 6 months after infarction, the dilatation was compensatory such that stroke volumes and cardiac outputs at rest and during exercise were relatively preserved, albeit with greater utilization of the Starling's mechanism during exercise (Fig. 3.6).

With longer follow-up, however, at 1.5 and 3 years, the submaximal exercise stroke volumes were grossly inadequate despite further dilatation and increased left ventricular filling pressure. It is important

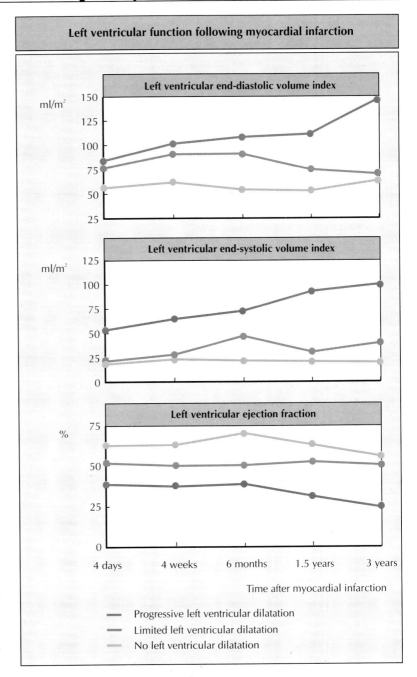

Fig. 3.5. Changes in left ventricular volumes and ejection fractions during 3-year follow-up of patients after myocardial infarction. The patients were subdivided into three groups: those with progressive dilatation (in whom EDVI rose by >8% at each measurement), those with limited dilatation (in whom EDVI did not continue to increase after 6 months) and those with no dilatation (in whom EDVI did not exceed 8% above baseline). Published by permission [72].

to note that the haemodynamic deterioration was not due to progression of coronary artery disease or further infarction. The progressive deterioration was considered to be due to diminished function of regions with 'normal' wall motion. Remarkably, the dilatative process progressed over the 3 years of follow-up, but left ventricular volumes and ejection fractions were seen to deviate most from the initial values during measurements at the later stages (1.5 and 3 years)

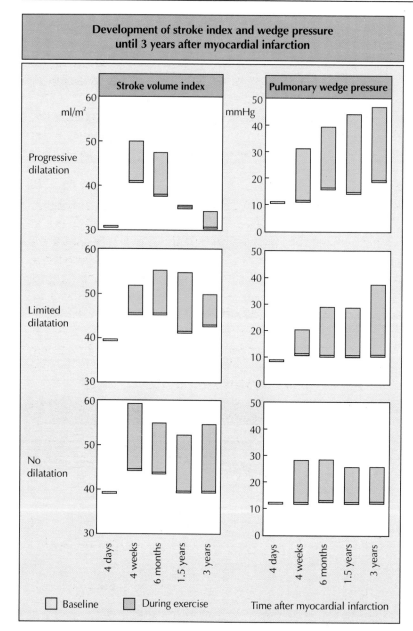

Fig. 3.6. The development of stroke index and mean pulmonary capillary wedge pressure until 3 years after myocardial infarction. Measurements of patients with progressive, limited and no dilatation are given at baseline and during supine bicycle exercise at 50 W. Except for stroke index with progressive dilatation at 1.5 and 3 years, all values were significantly higher during exercise than at baseline. Published by permission [72].

(Fig. 3.5). This finding of progressive ventricular dilatation and dysfunction may be secondary to on-going cardiomyocyte necrosis and replacement fibrosis described above.

If we postulate that the progressive cardiomyocyte loss leading to further dysfunction is due to prolonged activation of the sympathetic system and RAS, the next question is whether ACE inhibition after sizeable myocardial infarction can prevent the progressive deterioration in cardiac function. Schoemaker and colleagues [73] showed that this is possible in a rat model of moderately large infarction. Interestingly, they also observed that improvement in cardiac function was observed only 'when treatment was started after completion of the healing process' whereas 'early treatment not only failed to improve ventricular function, but may have a deleterious effect on the heart'.

There has been no study on the impact of ACE inhibition on cardiac functional capacity in patients after myocardial infarction. Serial measurements of left ventricular volumes have been conducted only using echocardiography [74,75] which is by no means an ideal tool to measure ventricular volumes. In a substudy of the Survival and Ventricular Enlargement (SAVE) trial, St John-Sutton and colleagues showed that captopril attenuates left ventricular dilatation in the subgroup without subsequent adverse cardiovascular events, for example further myocardial infarction [76]. The extents of ventricular enlargement in those who suffered adverse cardiovascular events were the same whether treated with captopril or placebo (Fig. 3.7). This finding can be reconciled with the concept that once myocardial infarction has occurred, compensatory ventricular dilatation is inexorable, with or without ACE inhibition, whereas ACE inhibition may attenuate ventricular dilatation by preventing on-going myocyte loss in the absence of further myocardial infarction.

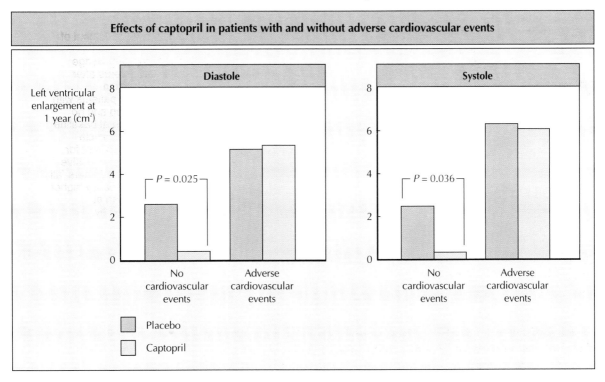

Fig. 3.7. Changes in left ventricular area between baseline and 1 year in patients with and without adverse cardiovascular events treated either with placebo or captopril. Published by permission [76].

Physiological versus pathological remodelling: a fine balance

Activation of neuroendocrine and local tissue systems serves to stimulate the reparative processes after myocardial infarction but overstimulation tends to overload the ventricles and exacerbate dysfunction and infarct expansion. Consequently, it can be seen that any intervention to limit the damage caused by overstimulation must be tailored to prevent oversuppression of the reparative response.

Given what we know of the temporal sequence of neurohormone-stimulated events after myocardial infarction, it seems that the key to achieving the optimum therapeutic balance lies in the timing of any interventions. For example, institution of ACE inhibition too soon after myocardial infarction is likely to inhibit necessary wound-healing processes, further compromising ventricular dysfunction. Delayed introduction would allow the initial healing to occur but then minimize the subsequent detrimental effects on the myocardium of catecholamines and angiotensin II, thus reducing the progression of ventricular dysfunction.

Further discussion of this premise can be found in Chapters 4 and 5, which examine the evidence from clinical trials of ACE inhibition after myocardial infarction in humans and the lessons for clinical practice from those trials, respectively.

References

1. Hutchins GM, Bulkley BH: **Infarct expansion versus extension: two different complications of acute myocardial infarction.** *Am J Cardiol* 1978, **41**:1127–1132.

2. Weisman HF, Healy B: **Myocardial infarct expansion, infarct extension and reinfarction: pathophysiologic concepts.** *Prog Cardiovasc Dis* 1987, **30**:73–110.

3. Eaton LW, Weiss JL, Bulkely BH, *et al.*: **Regional cardiac dilatation after acute myocardial infarction. Recognition by two-dimensional echocardiography.** *N Engl J Med* 1979, **300**:57–62.

4. Erlebacher JA, Weiss JL, Eaton LW, *et al.*: **Late effects of acute infarct dilation on heart size: a two dimensional echocardiographic study.** *Am J Cardiol* 1982, 49:1120–1126.

5. Schuster EH, Bulkley BH: **Expansion of transmural myocardial infarction: a pathophysiologic factor in cardiac rupture.** *Circulation* 1979, **60**:1532–1538.

6. Jugdutt BI, Michorowski BL: **Role of infarct expansion in rupture of the ventricular septum after acute myocardial infarction. A two-dimensional echocardiographic study.** *Clin Cardiol* 1987, **10**:641–652.

7. Mitchell GF, Lamas GA, Vaughan DE, Pfeffer MA: **Infarct expansion does not contribute to late left ventricular enlargement [abstract].** *Circulation* 1989, **80** (suppl II):II589.

8. Mitchell GF, Lamas GA, Vaughan DE, Pfeffer MA: **Changes in local curvature accompany left ventricular enlargement following anterior myocar-**

dial infarction [abstract]. *J Am Coll Cardiol* 1990, **15**:15A.

9. Fishbein MC, MacLean D, Maroko PR: **The histologic evolution of myocardial infarction.** Chest 1978, **73**:843–849.

10. Vracko R, Thorning D, Frederickson RG: **Connective tissue cells in healing rat myocardium.** *Am J Pathol* 1989, **134**:993–1006.

11. Parmley WW Chuuck L, Kivowitz C, *et al.*: *In vitro* **length-tension relations of human ventricular aneurysms.** *Am J Cardiol* 1973, **32**: 889–894.

12. Bulkley BH, Roberts WC: **Steroid therapy during acute myocardial infarction: a cause of delayed healing and of ventricular aneurysm.** *Am J Med* 1974, **56**:211–250.

13. Jugdutt BI, Basualdo CA: **Myocardial infarct expansion during indomethacin or ibuprofen therapy for symptomatic post infarction pericarditis: influence of other pharmacologic agents during remodelling.** *Can J Cardiol* 1989, **5**:211– 221.

14. Brown EJ, Kloner RA, Schoen FJ, *et al.*: **Scar thinning due to ibuprofen administration after experimental myocardial infarction.** *Am J Cardiol* 1983, **51**: 877–883.

15. Hammerman H, Kloner RA, Schoen FJ, *et al.*: **Indomethacin-induced scar thinning after experimental myocardial infarction.** *Circulation* 1983, **67**:1290–1295.

16. Hammerman H, Schoen FJ, Braunwald E, Kloner RA: **Drug-induced expansion of infarct: Morphologic and functional correlations.** *Circulation* 1984, **69**:611– 617.

17. Jugdutt BI: **Delayed effects of early infarct-limiting therapies on healing after myocardial infarction.** *Circulation* 1985, **72**:904–914.

18. Brilla C, Janicki JS, Weber KT: **Cardioreparative effects of lisinopril in rats with genetic hypertension and left ventricular hypertrophy.** *Circulation* 1991, **83**:1771–1779.

19. Brilla C, Janicki JS, Weber KT: **Impaired diastolic function and coronary reserve in genetic hypertension. Role of interstitial fibrosis and medial thickening of intramyocardial coronary arteries.** *Circ Res* 1991, **69**:107–115.

20. Weber KT, Janicki JS: **The heart as a muscle pump system and the concept of heart failure.** *Am Heart J* 1979, **98**:371–384.

21. Pfeffer MA, Braunwald E: **Ventricular remodelling after myocardial infarction: experimental observations and clinical implications.** *Circula-*tion 1990, **81**:1161–1172.

22. Pfeffer MA: **Ventricular remodelling and expansion after myocardial infarction.** In *Myocardial Infarction* edited by Gersh B, Rahimtolo FH. Chapman and Hall, 1991.

23. Tan LB, Jalil JE, Pick R, Janicki JS, Weber KT: **Cardiac myocyte necrosis induced by angiotensin II.** *Circ Res* 1991, **69**:1185–1195.

24. McDonald L, Baker C, Bray C, McDonald A, Restieaux N: **Plasma catecholamines after cardiac infarction.** *Lancet* 1969, **ii**:1021–1023.

25. Nabel E, Topol E, Galeana A, *et al.*: **A randomized placebo-controlled trial of combined early intravenous captopril and recombinant tissue-type plaminogen activator therapy in acute myocardial infarction.** *J Am Coll Cardiol* 1991, **17**:467–473.

26. Sigurdsson A, Held P, Swedberg K: **Short and long-term neurohormonal activation following acute myocardial infarction.** *Am Heart J* 1993, **126**:1068–1076.

27. McAlpine H, Morton J, Leckie B, Rumley A, Gillen G, Dargie HJ: **Neuroendocrine activation after myocardial infarction.** *Br Heart J* 1988, **60**:117–124.

28. McMurray J, Lang C, MacLean D, McDevitt D, Struthers A: **Neuroendocrine changes post myocardial infarction: effects of xamoterol.** *Am Heart J* 1990, **120**:56–62.

29. Vaughan D, Lamas G, Pfeffer MA: **Role of left ventricular dysfunction in selective neurohumoral activation in the recovery of anterior wall acute myocardial infarction.** *Am J Cardiol* 1990, **66**:529–532.

30. Rouleau J, Moye L, de Champlain J, *et al.*: **Activation of neurohumoral systems following acute myocardial infarction.** *Am J Cardiol* 1991, **68**:80D–86D.

31. Kunapuli SP, Kumar A: **Molecular cloning of human angiotensinogen cDNA and evidence for presence of its mRNA in rat heart.** *Circ Res* 1987, **60**:786–790.

32. Dzau VJ, Ingelfinger J, Pratt RE, Ellison KE: **Identification of messenger RNA sequence in mouse and rat brains.** *Hypertension* 1986, **86**:544–548.

33. Paul M, Wagner D, Metzger R, Ganten D, Lang RE, Suzuki F, Murakami K, Burbach JHP, Ludwig G: **Quantification of renin mRNA in various mouse tissues by a novel solution hybridization assay.** *J Hypertens* 1988, **6**:247–252.

34. Schunkert H, Dzau V, Tang SS, Hirsch AT, Apstein CS, Lorell BH: **Increased rat cardiac angiotensin converting enzyme activity and mRNA expression in pressure overload left ventricular hypertrophy.** *J Clin Invest* 1990, **86**:1913–1920.

35. Lindpaintner K, Jin M, Nidermaier N, Wilhelm MJ, Ganten D: **Cardiac angiotensinogen and its local activation in the isolated perfused beating heart.** *Circ Res* 1990, **67**:564–573.

36. Mukherjee A, Kulkarni PV, Haghani Z, Sutko JL: **Identification and characterization of angiotensin II receptors in cardiac sarcolemma.** *Biochem Biophys Res Commun* 1982, **105**:575–581.

37. Wright GB, Alexander RW, Ekstein LS, Gimbrone MA: **Characterization of the rabbit ventricular myocardial receptor for angiotensin II.** *Mol Pharmacol* 1983, **24**:213–221.

38. Baker KM, Campanile CP, Trachte GI, Peach MJ: **Identification and characterization of the rabbit angiotensin II myocardial receptor.** *Circ Res* 1984, **54**:286–293.

39. Baker KM, Singer HA: **Identification and characterization of guinea pig angiotensin II ventricular and atrial receptors: coupling to inositol phosphate production.** *Circ Res* 1988, **62**:896–904.

40. Urata H, Healy B, Stewart RW, Bumpus FM, Husain A: **Angiotensin II receptors in normal and failing hearts.** *J Clin Endocrinol Metab* 1989, **69**:54–66.

41. Allen AM, Yamada H, Mendelsohn FAO: ***In vitro autoradiographic localization of binding to angiotensin receptors in the rat heart.*** *Int J Cardiol* 1990, **28**:25–33.

42. Rogg H, Schmid A, Gasparo M: **Identification and characterization of angiotensin II receptor subtypes in rabbit ventricular myocardium.** *Biochem Biophys Res Commun* 1990, **173**:416–422.

43. Sechi LA, Griffin CA, Grady EF, Kalinyak JE, Schambelan M: **Characterization of angiotensin II receptor subtypes in rat heart.** *Circ Res* 1992, **71**:1482–1489.

44. Robertson AL, Khairallah PA: **Angiotensin II: Rapid localization in nuclei of smooth and cardiac muscle.** *Science* 1971, **172**:1138–1139.

45. Re RN, Macphee AA, Fallon JT: **Specific nuclear binding of angiotensin II by rat liver and spleen nuclei.** *Clin Sci* 1981, **61**:245–247.

46. Re RN, Vizard DL, Brown J, Bryan SE: **Angiotensin II receptors in chromatin fragments generated by micrococcal nuclease.** *Biochem Biophys Res Commun* 1984, **119**:220–227.

47. Muellerleile MR, Lunzer MM, Judd D, Dizon FD, Jones MB, Hirsch AT: **Activation of the cardiac renin–angiotensin system in response to sodium restriction [abstract 728-4].** *J Am Coll Cardiol* 1994, 1A-484A.

48. Baker KM, Chernin MI, Wixson SK, Aceto JA: **Renin–angiotensin system involvement in pressure overloaded cardiac hypertrophy in rats.** *Am J Physiol* 1990, **259**:H324–H332.

49. Lorell BH, Schunkert H, Grice WN, Tang WN, Apstein CS, Dzau VJ: **Alteration in cardiac angiotensin converting enzyme activity in pressure overload hypertrophy.** *Circulation* 1989, **80** (suppl 2):459–1323.

50. Schunkert H, Jackson B, Tang SS, *et al.*: **Distribution and functional significance of cardiac angiotensin converting enzyme in hypertrophied rat hearts.** *Circulation* 1993, **87**:1328–1339.

51. Fabris B, Jackson B, Kohzuki M, Perich R, Johnston CI: **Increased cardiac angiotensin-converting enzyme in rats with chronic heart failure.** *Clin Exp Pharmacol Physiol* 1990, **17**:309–314.

52. Finckh M, Hellman W, Ganten D, *et al.*: **Enhanced angiotensinogen gene expression and angiotensin converting enzyme activity in tachypacing-induced heart failure in rats.** *Basic Res Cardiol* 1991, **86**:303–316.

53. Jackson TR, Blair LAC, Marshall J, Goedert M, Hanley MR: **The *mas* oncogene encodes an angiotensin receptor.** *Nature* 1988, **335**:437–440.

54. Khairallah PA, Kanabus J: **Angiotensin and myocardial protein synthesis.** In *Perspectives in Cardiovascular Research* Vol 8 edited by Tarazi RC, Dunbar JB. New York: Raven Press, 1983, pp 337–347.

55. Brilla CG, Zhou G, Matsubara L, Weber KT: **Collagen metabolism in cultured adult cardiac fibroblasts: response to angiotensin and aldosterone.** *J Mol Cell Cardiol* 1994, **26**:809–820.

56. Benjamin IJ, Jalil JE, Tan LB, Cho K, Weber KT, Clark WA: **Isoproterenol-induced myocardial fibrosis in relation to myocyte necrosis.** *Circ Res* 1989, **65**:657–670.

57. Tan LB, Benjamin IJ, Clark WA: **Beta-adrenergic receptor desensitization may serve a cardioprotective role.** *Cardiovasc Res* 1992, **26**:608–614.

58. Volders PGA, Willems IEMG, Cleutjens JPM, Arends J-W, Havenith MG, Daemen MJAP: **Interstitial collagen is increased in the non-infarcted human myocardium after myocardial infarction.**

J Mol Cell Cardiol 1993, **25**:1317–1323.

59. Beltrami CA, Finato N, Rocco M, *et al.*: **Structural basis of end-stage failure in ischemic cardiomyopathy in humans.** *Circulation* 1994, **89**:151–163.

60. Michel J-B, Lattion A-L, Salzmann J-L, De Lourdes Cerol M, Camilleri J-P, Corvol P: **Hormonal and cardiac effects of converting enzyme inhibition in rat myocardial infarction.** *Circ Res* 1988, **62**:641–650.

61. van Krimpen, Schoemaker RG, Cleujens JP, *et al.*: **Angiotensin I converting enzyme inhibitors and cardiac remodelling.** *Basic Res Cardiol* 1991, **86** (suppl 1):149–155.

62. Judd JT, Wexler BC: **Prolyl hydroxylase and collagen metabolism after experimental myocardial infarction.** *Am J Physiol* 1975, **228**:212–216.

63. Jugdutt BI, Amy RWM: **Healing after myocardial infarction in the dog: changes in infarct hydroxyproline and topography.** *J Am Coll Cardiol* 1986, **7**:91–102.

64. Tan LB: **Evaluation of cardiac dysfunction, cardiac reserve and inotrophic response.** *Postgrad Med J* 1991, **67** (suppl 1):S10–S20.

65. Jackson B, Mendelsohn FAO, Johnston CI: **Angiotensin converting enzyme inhibition: prospects for the future.** *J Cardiovasc Pharmacol* 1991, **18** (suppl 7):S4–S8.

66. Hirsch AT, Talsness CE, Schunkert H, Paul M, Dzau VJ: **Tissue-specific activation of cardiac angiotensin coverting enzyme in experimental heart failure.** *Circ Res* 1991, **69**:475–482.

67. Reiss K, Capassa JM, Huang H-E, Meggs LG, Li P, Anversa P: **ANG II receptors, c-*myc* and c-*jun* in myocytes after myocardial infarction and ventricular failure.** *Am J Physiol* 1993, **264**:H760–H769.

68. Lindpaintner K, Lu W, Niedermajer J, Schieffer B, Just H, Ganten D, Drexler H: **Selective activation of cardiac angiotensinogen gene expression in post-infarction ventricular remodelling in the rat.** *J Mol Cell Cardiol* 1993, **25**:133–143.

69. Pfeffer JM, Pfeffer MA, Braunwald E: **Influence of chronic captopril therapy on the infarcted left ventricle of the rat.** *Circ Res* 1985, **57**:84–95.

70. Gay RG: **Early and late effects of captopril treatment after large myocardial infarction in rats.** *J Am Coll Cardiol* 1990, **16**:967–977.

71. Pfeffer MA, Pfeffer JM, Steinberg C, Finn P: **Survival after an experimental myocardial infarction: beneficial effects of long-term therapy with captopril.** *Circulation* 1985, **72**:406–412.

72. Gaudron P, Eiles C, Kugler I, Ertl G: **Progressive left ventricular dysfunction and remodeling after myocardial infarction. Potential mechanisms and early predictors.** *Circulation* 1993, **87**:755–763.

73. Schoemaker RG, Debets JJM, Struyker Boudier HAJ, Smits JFM: **Delayed but not immediate captopril therapy improves cardiac function in conscious rats, following myocardial infarction.** *J Mol Cell Cardiol* 1991, **23**:187197.

74. Sharpe N, Smith H, Murphy J, Hannan S: **Treatment of patients with symptomless left ventricular dysfunction after myocardial infarction.** *Lancet* 1988, **i**:255–259.

75. Sharpe N, Smith H, Murphy J, Greaves S, Hart H, Gamble G: **Early prevention of left ventricular dysfunction after myocardial infarction with angiotensin-converting-enzyme inhibition.** *Lancet* 1991, **337**:872–876.

76. St John-Sutton MG, Pfeffer MA, Plappert T, *et al.*: **Quantitative two-dimensional echocardiographic measurements are major predictors of adverse cardiovascular events after acute myocardial infarction. The protective effects of captopril.** *Circulation* 1994, **89**:68–75.

77. Farrer-Brown G: *A Colour Atlas of Cardiac Pathology.* London: Wolfe Medical Publications Ltd, 1977.

4

Data from clinical trials of ACE inhibition after myocardial infarction

Acute myocardial infarction leaves survivors at increased risk of fatal and non-fatal cardiovascular events. After myocardial infarction, systolic and diastolic function are compromised; prognosis is related to the size and location of the infarct, which strongly influences the severity of the left ventricular dysfunction and resultant complications. As has been discussed in the preceding chapters, the non-infarcted viable myocardium maintains the function of the cardiac pump as far as possible: left ventricular remodelling of the infarcted area and ventricular dilatation are initially an adaptive response to maintain cardiac output and blood pressure. The sympatho-adrenal and renin–angiotensin systems seem paramount in mediating these effects.

In patients with no subsequent clinical evidence of left ventricular dysfunction, the activation of the sympatho-adrenal and renin–angiotensin systems in response to a myocardial infarction subsides by about the third day after infarction [1]. In patients with overt cardiac dysfunction, however, both systems remain activated. Given that the first group of patients have a better survival prospect than the second, on-going overactivation of the neurohormonal mechanisms may be a marker of damage or indeed a cause of further damage, whereas the initial response could be an important protective response to maintain function. This is not a universally accepted view; some recent thinking appears to assume all cardiac remodelling and neurohormonal activation to be harmful in all patients at all times and that it should be counteracted. This has led to trials involving some 150 000 patients to assess strategies aimed at blocking this activation. We subscribe to the view that the primary objective in treating patients who have had a myocardial infarction is to allow the healing response and repair processes that occur in the immediate and early aftermath of a myocardial infarction to do so unimpeded. This may involve allowing some compensatory remodelling (hypertrophy and dilatation) to occur. By adjusting the timing of interventions to reduce deleterious neurohormonal activation, for example, ACE inhibition, it is possible to maintain myocardial viability both immediately and in the long term. We base this view on our interpretation of the results of recent large-scale clinical trials of ACE inhibition after myocardial infarction and earlier small-scale studies in humans.

Rationale for large-scale clinical trials of ACE inhibition after myocardial infarction

The evidence from animal studies that ventricular remodelling after induced myocardial infarction was attenuated by administration of an ACE inhibitor (see Chapter 3) and the known high risk associated with enlarged end-systolic or end-diastolic volumes [2] prompted a series of similar investigation in humans to see whether ACE inhibition attenuated the progressive increases in ventricular volume seen in some patients after myocardial infarction.

In a randomized, double-blind, placebo-controlled trial, Pfeffer and colleagues [3,4] examined the effect of captopril on progressive ventricular dilatation after anterior myocardial infarction in 59 patients with a ventricular ejection fraction of 45% or less. Treatment with captopril was initiated on average 20 days after myocardial infarction (range 11–31 days). After 1 year, left ventricular end-diastolic volumes had not increased significantly in the captopril-treated group compared with baseline volumes in this group, and left ventricular filling pressures were decreased ($P < 0.01$). A subset of 38 men without limitation attributed to ischaemic chest pain on exercise completed four exercise tests at 3-month intervals. In these men, exercise capacity, again compared with baseline (a notoriously dubious form of analysis), was consistently increased in those given captopril compared with the placebo group ($P < 0.05$). This attenuating effect of captopril was reported to be more marked in patients with persistent occlusion of the left anterior descending artery at baseline.

It is important to note that the patient group in this study is a highly selected one and that this restricts the conclusions that can be drawn from it, especially given the caveats covering the 'before and after' method of analysis. The changes in volume were small and the appropriate analysis comparing change in volume with captopril versus placebo was not undertaken. The applicability of these findings to clinical practice was therefore uncertain.

A similar study was carried out by Sharpe and colleagues [5] but with some important differences. They randomized 60 patients with left ventricular ejection fractions of less than 45% but without clinical evidence of heart failure 1 week after Q-wave infarction to three groups: captopril 25 mg thrice daily, frusemide 40 mg daily, or placebo. No patient had undergone thrombolytic therapy and those requiring treatment for ischaemic heart disease, heart failure or arrhythmias were excluded. Left ventricular volumes (as measured by cross-sectional echocardiography, a notoriously difficult and potentially inaccurate method) increased significantly in the placebo and frusemide-treated groups during the 12 months of the trial ($P < 0.05$) and decreased in the captopril-treated group. At baseline, however, the captopril group have higher end-diastolic volumes, and there was little difference in absolute volumes between the three groups at 1 year.

Sharpe and colleagues subsequently speculated that greater benefit might have been observed if captopril treatment had been started earlier than 1 week, given that substantial ventricular dilatation had already occurred by then. They tested this hypothesis in a later study [6] in which captopril 50 mg twice daily was given to patients who had suffered a Q-wave infarction 24–48 hours, rather than 1 week, after infarct. In this instance, more than two-thirds of patients had received thrombolytic therapy. Changes in end-diastolic and end-systolic volumes and ejection fractions as assessed by serial echocardiography were qualitatively similar to the 1988 study, indicating a beneficial effect of captopril. Even by the time of the first echo measurement there was a substantial increase in systolic and diastolic dimensions compared with normal values. Again, however, the captopril group had higher end-systolic and end-diastolic volumes at baseline.

Comparison of the relative volume changes observed in these studies led the authors to conclude that administration of an ACE inhibitor was both feasible and likely to result in treatment benefit. These studies cannot, however, separate changes in the lengths of the infarcted segments from increases in size of the ventricle as part of an appropriate compensatory mechanism to maintain function. The observed changes were small and could not be assumed to indicate benefit. The relationship between these volume changes to the functional capacity of the heart and to the prognosis of the patients is unclear.

A large-scale clinical trial with mortality as the endpoint was therefore needed to assess the role for ACE inhibitors in the treatment of patients after a myocardial infarction.

The trials conducted to date to address this issue can be grouped according to their design: that is, whether they recruited a selected patient population or not, whether ACE inhibition was initiated soon after myocardial infarction (within 24–36 hours of infarct) or later (3–14 days after infarct), and whether treatment and follow-up were long-term or not. It is important to take these factors into account when drawing conclusions from the results of the trials and we have chosen to present our discussion here using these groupings.

Non-selective early-intervention trials

Second Cooperative North Scandinavian Enalapril Survival Study (CONSENSUS II)

The first published early-intervention trial to examine the hypothesis that early ACE inhibition after myocardial infarction improves long-term survival was the second Cooperative North Scandinavian Enalapril Survival Study (CONSENSUS II) [7]. It was based on the premise that infarct expansion and ventricular dilatation occur soon after the onset of infarction, and the earlier the off-loading effects on the ventricle can be achieved using intravenous enalaprilat, the more effective can be the prevention of ventricular dilatation. This was expected to be translated into better preservation of ventricular function and therefore survival benefits. Six thousand and ninety patients with suspected myocardial infarction and blood pressures over 100/60 mmHg were randomized to either placebo or intravenous enalaprilat followed by oral enalapril initiated within 24 hours of onset of acute infarction. All patients also received standard therapy. The primary endpoint was all-cause mortality at 6 months; secondary endpoints were 1-month mortality, effect of treatment on cause of death, reinfarction and worsening heart failure.

CONSENSUS II

- 6090 patients with suspected acute myocardial infarction

- Enalapril versus placebo given within 24 hours of acute myocardial infarction

- Primary endpoint = all-cause mortality at 6 months. Prematurely ended because of excess mortality in the enalapril group

The safety committee monitoring the trial recommended changes to the protocol after 8 months because of a non-significant trend towards increased mortality among patients with early hypotensive reactions to enalapril: the minimal blood pressure for recruitment was raised to 105/65 mmHg and the duration of infusion of enalaprilat was increased to 3 hours. Furthermore, they required that the infusion be stopped and not restarted if systolic blood pressure fell to below 100 mmHg, or by more than 30 mmHg, or diastolic blood pressure to below 60 mmHg.

One year into the trial, the safety committee recommended that the trial be stopped because of the high probability that the null hypothesis (that enalapril was no better than placebo) would apply and because of concern about a possible adverse effect of enalapril among elderly patients with early hypotensive reactions [8].

By the end of the trial, 598 patients had died: 286 in the placebo group and 312 in the enalapril group (a difference of 26 deaths; $P = 0.26$). Cumulative mortality rates are shown in Figure 4.1. One hundred and thirty-two of the enalapril deaths were classified as being due to progressive heart failure compared with 104 in the placebo group, a difference of 28 deaths. This suggests that most of the excess mortality in the enalapril group was due to progressive cardiac failure. Given that the rationale for the trial and findings from previous studies in animals and humans suggested that the survival benefit of ACE inhibitors was likely to be as a result of an improvement in pump function, this result was unexpected.

There are a number of possible explanations for these findings:
- The reported effects of ACE inhibitors on left ventricular dilatation may not translate into improvement in survival (but later studies indicate that it does).
- The dose of enalapril may have been inadequate, although the target oral dose (reached in 82% of patients) was similar to the dose given for heart failure in trials that demonstrated a reduction in mortality [9,10].
- The lack of beneficial effect could be due to the timing of administration of enalapril. Early after infarction, myocardial protein synthesis stimulated by angiotensin II and catecholamines stimulates myocyte growth and collagen synthesis which, in the short term, serve to maintain cardiac structural integrity and normalize cardiac performance. This healing process may be

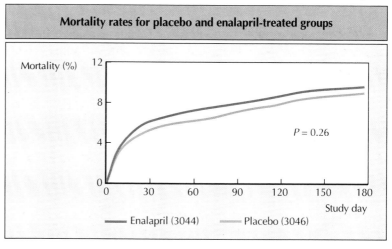

Fig 4.1. Kaplan–Meier life-table mortality curves for the placebo and enalapril-treated group from CONSENSUS II. Published by permission [7].

suppressed by early ACE inhibition, thus worsening clinical outcome. There is some evidence from animal studies to support this: Schoemaker and colleagues [11] found that captopril administered to rats soon after myocardial infarction did not improve cardiac reserve during follow-up but, when given later, cardiac reserve was improved.

- A reduction in coronary perfusion pressure caused by systemic hypotension in response to intravenous enalaprilat may have led to an increase in subendocardial ischaemia, and subsequently to increased mortality. However, the design of the study does not allow assessment of the impact of early hypotension on the excess mortality, but only speculation.

Gruppo Italiano per lo Studio della Sopravvivenza nell'Infarto Miocardio (GISSI)-3 study

The recently published trial from the Gruppo Italiano per lo Studio della Sopravvivenza nell'Infarto Miocardio (GISSI) [12] examined the effects of lisinopril and nitrate therapy, initiated within 24 hours of infarction, on the mortality and morbidity of patients with suspected myocardial infarction in a multicentre, randomized, open (i.e. not blinded or placebo-controlled) trial. The primary endpoint was 6-week mortality; secondary endpoints were time to heart failure necessitating non-trial ACE inhibition or to death. Eligible patients presented within 24 hours of onset of symptoms and had no clear indications for or against the study treatments. Using a factorial design patients were randomly assigned oral lisinopril (10 mg once daily) for 6 weeks or open control as well as nitrates (intravenous nitrate initially followed by transdermal glyceryl trinitrate 10 mg once daily after 24 hours) or open control.

The authors report that lisinopril produced a small 0.8% reduction in absolute mortality from 7.1 to 6.3% (risk reduction 11%, 95% CI 1–21%; $2P = 0.03$). The survival curves of lisinopril-treated patients and controls separated early and continued to diverge throughout the six-week study period (Fig. 4.2). Lisinopril also reduced the rate of the other main outcome measure, the combined endpoint, from 17% of patients experiencing an event to 15.6%, a reduction of 1.4% (risk reduction 10%, 95% CI 2–16%; $2P = 0.009$). Administration of transdermal glyceryl trinitrate did not show any statistically significant independent effect on the same outcome measures (Fig. 4.2) but combined treatment with lisinopril and nitrates did produce a greater reduction in overall mortality (risk reduction 17%, 95% CI 3–30%)

GISSI-3

- 18 895 patients with suspected acute myocardial infarction

- Lisinopril versus placebo given within 24 hours of acute myocardial infarction

- Primary endpoint = all-cause mortality at 6 weeks

- Small statistically significant reduction (0.8%) in mortality in the lisinopril group

- Excess persistent hypotension (and subsequent death) in the lisinopril-treated group

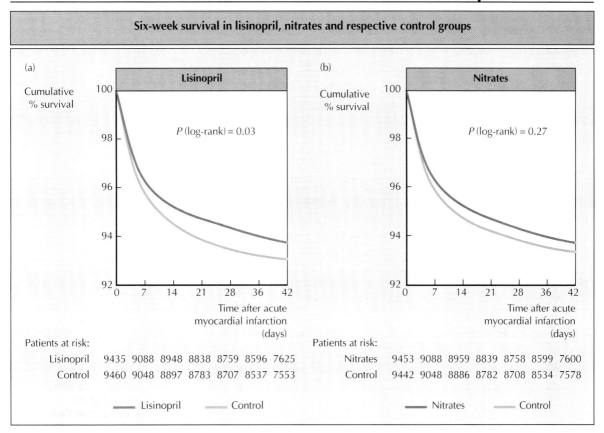

Fig 4.2. Survival curves for patients treated with lisinopril or nitrates and their control groups from the GISSI-3 study. Published by permission [12].

and the combined endpoint (risk reduction 15%, 95% CI 6–24%) than for lisinopril alone. The observed benefit with lisinopril was also seen in the pre-defined high-risk populations (elderly patients and women) for the combined endpoint.

The results and published interpretation of GISSI-3 bear close scrutiny. We know that patients experiencing myocardial infarction are not a homogeneous group and that those most likely to benefit from ACE inhibition are those with impaired ventricular function. Up to 5% of patients have severe heart failure after a myocardial infarction and a further 20% have some clinical evidence of heart failure complicating their presentation. On the evidence of CONSENSUS I and the Studies of Left Ventricular Dysfunction (SOLVD) treatment arm, we know that long-term ACE inhibition produces clear survival benefit for patients with heart failure, but not recent myocardial infarction. The Acute Infarction Ramipril Efficacy (AIRE) study [13] (see pp. 60–61) reported a survival benefit even at 30 days (risk reduction 29%; 95% CI –1–50%; $P = 0.053$) for patients selected on the basis of clinical evidence of heart failure (but excluding patients with severe heart failure) 2–9 days after a myocardial infarction and given ramipril. The reduction in mortality was considerably larger than that obtained in GISSI-3 over a comparable time scale and with almost identical risk as indicated by the 30-day mortality in the two groups.

By 6 months, the small mortality benefit seen in GISSI-3 had halved and was no longer significant. This contrasts with the AIRE study where, after an average follow-up of 15 months, there was a highly significant 27% reduction in mortality ($P = 0.002$). The duration of any mortality benefit is an important issue for those seeking to determine appropriate clinical practice on the basis of trial results.

It is quite possible that the bulk of the survival benefit in the lisinopril-treated group is concentrated in those patients who developed dysfunction, especially with severe failure, in the first few days after the index event. Patients in the GISSI-3 study were classified according to Killip status at randomization and a tenfold difference in the impact of lisinopril on mortality was observed according to Killip classification (three lives saved per 1000 patients treated in Killip class I versus 30 lives saved per 1000 patients in Killip class >I, i.e. more severe heart failure) [14]. Furthermore, it should be remembered that many of those in Killip class I–III would deteriorate to worse failure in the early period after infarction.

Data are presented on the incidence of adverse events in the trial groups in GISSI-3, an issue of some importance given the negative results of CONSENSUS II and the concerns about possible increased risk of death due to persistent hypotension in a subset of patients treated with an ACE inhibitor early after a myocardial infarction. The reported findings show that reinfarction, post-infarction angina, persistent hypotension, shock, renal dysfunction, stroke, the need for coronary artery bypass surgery and coronary angioplasty were all more common in the lisinopril-treated group, although only the excess in renal dysfunction and persistent hypotension were statistically significant. Persistent hypotension (defined as systolic blood pressure < 90 mmHg for more than one hour) occurred in 852 of the lisinopril group compared with 351 of the control group, an absolute excess number of hypotensive events attributable to lisinopril of 54 per 1000 patients treated. Within these two groups there were 145 and 102 deaths, respectively, giving an absolute excess of 43 deaths or 4.6 deaths per 1000 patients when treated with lisinopril. This excess is masked by a net reduction in the number of deaths observed for the trial as a whole (597 in the lisinopril group versus 673 in the control group: an absolute difference of only 76 deaths or a total of eight deaths prevented or delayed by treatment with lisinopril per 1000 patients). It is significant that the number of deaths prevented was greatest in the subgroup of patients who did not develop persistent hypotension (452 in the lisinopril group versus 571 in the control group; 12.6 deaths prevented or delayed by treatment with lisinopril per 1000 patients). As for CONSENSUS II the design of the study cannot resolve whether the excess hypotension produced by lisinopril had or did not have an adverse effect on mortality. Therefore, contrary to the authors' assertion that the use of lisinopril was 'remarkably safe', the immediate use of lisinopril in unselected patients after acute myocardial infarction may well produce harm in a subset of patients, while producing benefit in others. It does not appear to us that the GISSI-3 results allay the concerns over the early administration of ACE inhibition after myocardial infarction appropriately raised by CONSENSUS II, especially when the minor net benefit on mortality is even smaller and no longer significant at 6 months.

International Studies of Infarct Survival (ISIS)-4

The fourth International Studies of Infarct Survival (ISIS-4) was set up to compare the effect on survival of early administration of an oral preparation of captopril (within 24 hours of infarction) with placebo and with oral nitrates and intravenous magnesium. The study was under way when the results of CONSENSUS II were reported but the investigators decided to continue on the basis that use of a different class of ACE inhibitor as an oral preparation might have a different effect on survival [15].

All patients presenting within 24 hours of an acute myocardial infarction were considered eligible for inclusion in the study, unless there were clear indications for, or contraindications to, the trial therapies. Endpoints were 35-day and 6-month mortality.

The full results of the trial have not yet been published in the medical literature but initial findings were presented to the American Heart Association in November 1993 and released to the media at the same time. Nearly 60 000 patients were recruited into the study. Thirty-five-day mortality was reduced by 0.5% in the captopril group (6.78% versus 7.33% in the placebo group, $P = 0.04$). Six-month mortality was reduced by 0.6–0.7% ($P = 0.03$). The greatest benefits were seen

---

ISIS-4

- Nearly 60 000 patients with suspected acute myocardial infarction

- Captopril versus placebo within 24 hours of acute myocardial infarction

- Primary endpoints = 35-day and 6-month mortality

- Small, statistically significant reductions in mortality (35 days and 6 months) in the captopril group

in high-risk patients, although benefits of captopril treatment were present in all subgroups except those with a systolic blood pressure of less than 100 mmHg. A full assessment of the implications of this trial must await formal publication of the results, but the preliminary reports indicate to us, at least, that the survival benefit predominantly accrued to those patients with heart failure or likely substantial ventricular damage, for example, those with an anterior myocardial infarction.

Chinese CEI-AMI Clinical Trial Collaborative Group

This multicentre, double-blind, placebo-controlled trial was designed to investigate the effects of captopril (12.5 mg three times daily for 4 weeks) in patients with acute myocardial infarction within 36 hours of onset of symptoms. The target number of patients was 10 000. The primary end-point was mortality at 4 weeks, and secondary end-points were complications of infarction.

The results have not been published. Preliminary data indicate that 23–24% received thrombolysis, 72–75% aspirin and 57–60% calcium antagonists. Approximately 18% of patients had heart failure prior to entry into the study. Absolute mortality reduction was 0.3% at 4 weeks from 9.7% in the placebo group to 9.4% in the captopril group. The reduction was not statistically significant. The incidence of hypotension was higher in the captopril group (17.5% versus 10.7%).

Selective early-intervention trials

Survival of Myocardial Infarction Long-Term Evaluation (SMILE) study

The Survival of Myocardial Infarction Long-term Evaluation (SMILE) study [16] randomized 1556 patients to the ACE inhibitor zofenopril or placebo within 24 hours of myocardial infarction. The patients recruited were selected on the basis of a contraindication for thrombolytic therapy after an anterior myocardial infarction. The endpoints were death or refractory heart failure (i.e. heart failure uncontrolled by diuretics or digitalis) at 6 weeks. Six-week mortality was reduced in the zofenopril-treated group, but not significantly (8.3% with placebo versus 6.5% with zofenopril). A significant reduction was observed in the development of refractory heart failure at 6 weeks: 4.3% in the placebo group versus 2.2 % in the zofenopril

SMILE

- 1556 patients with acute myocardial infarction, thrombolytic therapy contraindicated

- Zofenopril versus placebo within 24 hours of acute myocardial infarction

- Primary endpoint = 6-week mortality or refractory heart failure at 6 weeks

group, a relative reduction of 49% ($P = 0.018$). The combined end-point also showed a statistically significant benefit in the zofenopril group with a relative risk reduction of 33% ($P = 0.008$).

At the time of the preliminary results being reported (September 1992), it was planned to continue the study as an open comparison of zofenopril and placebo to see whether the reduction in mortality became significant after one year. To date, these results have not been published.

The trend towards a survival benefit in this study contrasted with the negative trend seen in CONSENSUS II. It may be that the choice of ACE inhibitor and the mode of administration (non-sulphydryl versus sulphydryl; oral versus intravenous) accounts for the difference. We believe that it is more likely that the difference lies in the selection of patients; CONSENSUS II treated a largely unselected group of patients, most of whom received thrombolytic therapy before administration of an ACE inhibitor, whereas none of the SMILE patients had received thrombolytic therapy and all had evidence of anterior myocardial infarction. These patients are more likely to develop cardiac dysfunction. The preliminary results of ISIS-4 bear out this reasoning: greatest benefit was seen in the subset of patients who had an anterior infarct or who developed heart failure.

Captopril and Thrombolysis Study (CATS)

The Captopril and Thrombolysis Study (CATS) [17] randomized 298 patients with a first anterior myocardial infarction who had received streptokinase to either captopril (25 mg thrice daily) or placebo, within 6 hours of onset of symptoms.

Increase in ventricular volume over 3 months was modest (as shown in other post-infarct studies done since the introduction of routine thrombolysis [18]) and was not significantly reduced by captopril. The investigators concluded that any benefit of captopril in the first 3 months after myocardial infarction was likely to be by mechanisms other than attenuation of dilatation. Similar to the CONSENSUS II result, there was a non-significant excess of mortality (6% in the captopril group versus 4.7%) suggesting that very early administration of an ACE inhibitor after myocardial infarction is undesirable.

CATS

- 298 patients suffering a first acute myocardial infarction and given streptokinase

- Captopril versus placebo soon after acute myocardial infarction

- Primary endpoint = increase in ventricular volume

- No significant reduction by captopril

Selective delayed-intervention trials

Survival and Ventricular Enlargement (SAVE) study

The Survival and Ventricular Enlargement (SAVE) study [19] hypothesized that long-term administration of captopril to survivors of acute myocardial infarction who had baseline ventricular dysfunction (ejection fraction < 40%) but no symptoms of overt heart failure or myocardial ischaemia would reduce mortality and improve clinical outcome.

Two thousand two hundred and thirty-one patients recruited between 3 and 16 days (average day 11) after myocardial infarction on the basis of a radionuclide ejection fraction of 40% or less, and without evidence of active ischaemia (assessed by exercise test, coronary angiography or persistent chest pain), were randomized to captopril 75–150 mg daily or placebo. Patients were followed up for an average of 42 months.

At the end of the study, a 19% reduction in the risk of death from all causes was observed (95% CI 3–32; P = 0.019) in the captopril group compared with the placebo group (Fig. 4.3). The risk reduction in death from cardiovascular causes was 21% (95% CI 5–35; P = 0.014) for the captopril group. Within this group, there was a marked reduction in mortality due to progressive heart failure in the captopril

SAVE
• 2231 survivors of acute myocardial infarction with baseline ventricular dysfunction
• Captopril versus placebo within 3–16 days of acute myocardial infarction
• Primary endpoint = all-cause mortality at 42 months (average)

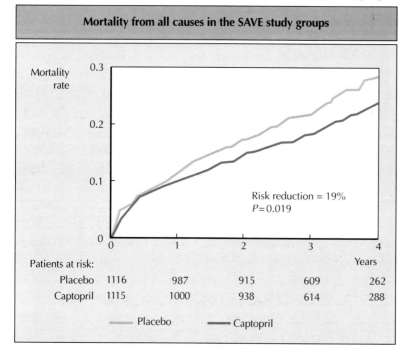

Fig 4.3. Cumulative mortality from all causes for the placebo and captopril-treated groups from SAVE. Published by permission [19].

group compared with the placebo group: a risk reduction of 36% (95% CI 4–58; P = 0.032)

The selection of patients for the SAVE study is important. Extensive measures were taken to exclude patients with detectable myocardial ischaemia: patients with a positive exercise test or persistent chest pain underwent coronary angiography (54% and 57% of the placebo and captopril groups, respectively) followed by revascularization if necessary. Furthermore, patients who experienced ischaemic discomfort with a test dose of captopril 6.25 mg were then excluded from the study analysis. Therefore, the SAVE study population was one of asymptomatic patients who could tolerate captopril and who did not have detectable myocardial ischaemia or in whom ischaemia had been corrected by coronary artery surgery or angioplasty.

The incidence of Q-wave acute myocardial infarction was high at 84% and only 33% of patients had undergone thrombolytic therapy. This compares with the CONSENSUS study population who had a much lower incidence of Q-wave infarctions (59%) and a higher incidence of patients receiving thrombolytic therapy (56%) [7]. Q-wave infarction and failure to administer thrombolytic therapy are both associated with persistent occlusion of the infarcted artery and so patients in the SAVE study were likely to have a greater tendency to progressive ventricular dilatation than those in the CONSENSUS study [20,21]. This may partly explain the positive results of SAVE compared with those of CONSENSUS; that is, the SAVE study appropriately selected those patients who were more likely to benefit from the test therapy.

It is also relevant to note that no clear survival benefit from captopril therapy was observed in the first 12 months of treatment (Fig. 4.3). Also, the incidence of myocardial infarction and congestive heart failure requiring open-label ACE inhibitor treatment or hospitalization was higher during the first 12 months than in the total study duration of 4 years. This may have negated the beneficial effects of captopril, as implied in a subsequently published SAVE substudy [22] which showed that, in patients who suffered adverse cardiovascular events, captopril did not confer protection against left ventricular enlargement.

Patients who have suffered a myocardial infarction are at risk from a number of different factors over the ensuing months and years: left ventricular dysfunction, ischaemic burden and tendency to develop arrhythmias. The SAVE study excluded patients who carried detectable ischaemic risk and those with overt cardiac failure at greatest risk from the effects of left ventricular impairment. It is therefore arguable how far the treatment benefit of captopril for the SAVE population can be extended to all patients suffering a myocardial infarction. It is even plausible that delaying the initiation of ACE inhibition until symptoms were present may have produced equivalent benefits and perhaps have avoided some early adverse events.

Acute Infarction Ramipril Efficacy (AIRE) study

The Acute Infarction Ramipril Efficacy (AIRE) [13] postulated that therapy with ramipril would lengthen survival of that subset of myocardial infarct patients who manifest clinical heart failure despite treatment with thrombolytic agents and aspirin and for whom beta blockers are relatively contraindicated. These patients are at particularly high risk as they have a propensity for fatal and non-fatal ischaemic, arrhythmic and haemodynamic events.

AIRE
• 2006 survivors of acute myocardial infarction with clinical signs of heart failure
• Ramipril versus placebo within 3–10 days of acute myocardial infarction
• Primary endpoint = all-cause mortality at 15 months (average)

Two thousand and six patients who had shown clinical evidence of heart failure at any time after an acute myocardial infarction were randomly allocated to double-blind treatment with either placebo (992 patients) or ramipril (1014 patients) 3–10 days after myocardial infarction. Patients with severe heart failure resistant to conventional therapy for whom ACE inhibition was considered mandatory were excluded. Follow-up was for a minimum of 6 months and an average of 15 months.

All-cause mortality (analysed on an intention-to-treat basis) was significantly lower for patients in the ramipril group (170 deaths; 17%) than for those in the placebo group (222 deaths; 23%) (Fig. 4.4.). The observed risk reduction was 27% (95% CI 11–40%; $P = 0.002$). Separation of the curves occurred early (as early as 30 days) and they continued to diverge throughout the study. The secondary endpoint was time to the first validated event (death, reinfarction, stroke or development of severe or resistant heart failure) and again the risk reduction for events in the ramipril group was highly statistically significant, at 19% (95% CI 5–31%; $P = 0.008$).

The observed benefit was consistent across different subgroups and was independent of the use of thrombolytic agents (given to 58% of patients), aspirin (given to 78% of patients) and beta blockers (given to 22% of patients).

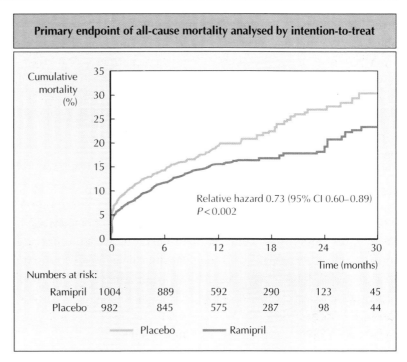

Primary endpoint of all-cause mortality analysed by intention-to-treat

Relative hazard 0.73 (95% CI 0.60–0.89)
$P < 0.002$

Numbers at risk:

Ramipril	1004	889	592	290	123	45
Placebo	982	845	575	287	98	44

Fig. 4.4. Mortality curves illustrating the primary endpoint of all-cause mortality analysed by intention-to-treat from the AIRE Study. Most patients were followed for less than 18 months and the curves were terminated at 30 months because of the small numbers of patients with prolonged follow-up. Published by permission [22].

The AIRE study was set up to take account of changing clinical practice and reflected a broad-based premise about the possible mechanisms of any clinical improvement produced by ACE inhibition after myocardial infarction: that appropriately timed ACE inhibition in a particular subset of patients at greatest risk of pathological left ventricular dilatation reduces the risk of subsequent adverse events. Included in this premise was the possibility that delayed ACE inhibition may be less deleterious to coronary perfusion (thus reducing subsequent ischaemic damage), may reduce the likelihood of developing arrhythmias, and may improve left ventricular haemodynamics. Clinicians participating in the trial were able to decide individually what they regarded as sufficiently severe heart failure unresponsive to conventional therapy to justify prescription of this group of drugs rather than inclusion in the AIRE study. The same criterion – clinical judgement – was also used in assessing the progression to severe or resistant heart failure for study patients necessitating, in the clinician's opinion, a switch from trial medication to open-label ACE inhibitor. No restrictions were imposed on therapy other than the use of ACE inhibitors. Thus, the results of the AIRE study can be taken to have a direct relevance to clinicians in that patients who are likely to benefit from treatment with ramipril after a myocardial infarction can be identified by simple, everyday measures.

The Trandolapril Cardiac Evaluation (TRACE) Study

An ongoing study of trandolapril (the Trandolapril Cardiac Evaluation Study, TRACE) [23] in reduced left ventricular function after myocardial infarction has selected patients on the basis of measured impaired ventricular function, as in SAVE, but, unlike in SAVE, patients with overt heart failure have not been excluded.

One thousand seven hundred and forty-nine patients with an ejection fraction below 35% as determined by echocardiography have been randomized to receive either placebo or trandolapril (4 mg daily), initiated between 2 and 7 days after acute myocardial infarction. Patients who could not tolerate a pre-trial oral test dose of 0.5 mg were excluded. Originally, the investigators planned to treat and follow up for 1 year but this has now been extended to 2 years since the publication of the SAVE results. We expect the results to be reported in late 1994.

TRACE
• 1749 survivors of acute myocardial infarction with reduced ventricular function or overt heart failure
• Trandolapril versus placebo within 2–7 days after acute myocardial infarction
• Primary endpoint = all-cause mortality
• Results not yet known

Interpretation of the trials

Large-scale trials inevitably include selected patients and give answers only to broad questions of treatment strategy. The clinician is faced with the individual patient and must use intelligent analysis of the trials to make the best decision. Patients who have severe damage to their ventricle after a myocardial infarction have a poor prognosis. Many will be receiving a diuretic and the need to start and continue ACE -inhibitor therapy is beyond question. If the ACE inhibitors had been convincingly shown to prevent re-infarction then justification for widespread treatment would be obvious. However, whatever evidence there is to support the role is as yet far from conclusive.

More difficult is to decide how wide to make the indications for ACE-inhibitor treatment and when to start therapy after myocardial infarction. The'mega-trials' also serve to highlight the question of how long treatment should be given since they tested a strategy of short-term, 4- to 6-week therapy. Patients with cardiogenic shock should not be given ACE inhibitors but those with severe failure and adequate blood pressure may on average benefit. However, those with critical narrowing of coronary vessels in whom vital perfusion depends on adequate perfusion pressure seem likely to be harmed by any agent which initially lowers blood pressure. On-going ischaemic pain, failing to resolve, would make many clinicians reluctant to prescribe ACE inhibitors.

References

1. Rouleau JL, Maye LA, de Champlain J, *et al.*: **Activation of neurohormonal systems following acute myocardial infarction.** *Am J Cardiol* 1991, **68**:80D–86D.
2. White HD, Norris RM, Brown MA, Brandt PWT, Whitlock RM, Wild CJ: **Left ventricular end systolic volume as the major determinant of survival after recovery from myocardial infarction.** *Circulation* 1987, **76**:44–51.
3. Pfeffer MA, Pfeffer JM, Steinberg C, Finn P: **Survival after experimental myocardial infarction: beneficial effects of long-term therapy with captopril.** *Circulation* 1985, **72**:406–412.
4. Pfeffer MA, Lamas GA, Vaughan DE, Parisi AF, Braunwald E: **Effect of captopril on progressive dilatation after anterior myocardial infarction.** *N Engl J Med* 1988, **319**:80–86.
5. Sharpe N, Smith H, Murphy J, Hannan S: **Treatment of patients with symptomless left ventricular dysfunction after mycocardial infarction.** *Lancet* 1988, **i**:255–259.
6. Sharpe N, Smith H, Murphy J, Greaves S, Hart H, Gamble G: **Early prevention of left ventricular dysfunction after myocardial infarction with angiotensin-converting-enzyme inhibition.** *Lancet* 1991, **337**:872–876.
7. Swedberg K, Held P, Kjekshus J, Rasmussen K, Rydén L, Wedel H [on behalf of the CONSENSUS II Study Group]: **Effects of the early administration of enalapril on mortality in patients with acute myocardial infarction. Result of the Cooperative North Scandinavian Enalapril Survival Study II (CONSENSUS II).** *N Engl J Med* 1992, **327**:678–684.
8. Furberg CD, Campbell RWF, Pi HB: **ACE inhibitors after myocardial infarction [letter].** *N Engl J Med* 1993, **328**:967–968.
9. SOLVD Investigators: **Effects of enalapril on survival in patients with reduced left ventricular ejection fractions and congestive heart failure.** *N Engl J Med* 1991, **325**:293–302.
10. SOLVD Investigators: **Effects of enalapril on mortality and the development of heart failure in asymptomatic patients with reduced ventricular ejection fractions.** *N Engl J Med* 1992, **327**:685–691.
11. Schoemaker RG, Debets JJM, Struker-Boudier HAJ, Smits JFM: **Delayed but not immediate captopril therapy improves cardiac function in conscious rats, following myocardial infarction.** *J Mol Cell Cardiol* 1991, **23**:187–197.
12. Gruppo Italiano per lo Studio della Sopravvivenza nell'Infarto Miocardio: **GISSI-3 effects of lisinopril and transdermal glyceryl trinitrate singly and together on 6-week mortality and ventricular function after acute myocardial infarction.** *Lancet* 1994, **343**:1115–1122.
13. Acute Infarction Ramipril Efficacy (AIRE) Study Investigators: **Effects of ramipril on mortality and morbidity of survivors of acute myocardial infarction with clinical evidence of heart failure.** *Lancet* 1993, **342**:821–828.
14. Tognoni G, on behalf of the Gruppo Italiano per lo Studio della Sopravvivenza nell'Infarto Miocardio: **ACE inhibitors after acute myocardial infarction.** *Lancet* 1994, **343**:1633–1634.
15. Fourth International Study of Infarct Survival Collaboration Group: **Protocol for a large simple study of the effects of oral mononitrate, of oral captopril and of intravenous magnesium: ISIS-4.** *Am J Cardiol* 1991, **68**:87D–100D.
16. Ambrosioni E for the SMILE Study Working Party: **Survival of myocardial infarction long-term evaluation (SMILE).** *Scrip No. 1753*, 1992, p. 29. **check for full authors**
17. Van Gilst W for the CATS Working Party: **Captopril and thrombolysis study.** *Scrip No 1753* 1992, p. 29.
18. Gaudron P, Gilles C, Kugler I, Ertle G: **Progressive left ventricular dysfunction and remodelling after myocardial infarction. Potential mechanisms and early predictions.** *Circulation* 1993, **87**:755–763.
19. Pfeffer MA, Braunwald E, Moyé LA, *et al.*: **Effect of captopril on mortality and morbidity in patients with left ventricular dysfunction after myocardial infarction. Results of the Survival and Ventricular Enlargement Trial.** *N Engl J Med* 1992, **327**:669–677.
20. Jugdutt BI, Tang SB, Khan MI, Basualdo CA: **Functional impact of remodelling during healing after non-Q-wave versus Q-wave anterior myocardial infarction in the dog.** *J Am Coll Cardiol* 1992, **20**:722–731.
21. Lamas GA, Pfeffer MA, Braunwald E: **Patency of the infarct-related coronary artery and ventricular geometry.** *Am J Cardiol* 1991, **68**:41D–51D.

22. St John Sutton MG, Pfeffer MA, Plappert T, *et al.*: **Quantitative two-dimensional echocardiographic measurements are major predictors of adverse cardiovascular events after acute myocardial infarction. The protective effects of captopril.** *Circulation* 1994, **89**:68–75.

23. The TRACE Study Group: **The TRAndolapril Cardiac Evaluation (TRACE) Study: Rationale, design and baseline characteristics of the screened population.** *Am J Cardiol* 1994, **73**:44C–50C.

5

Clinical implications of the mega-trial data

Basic science research provides ways of elucidating mechanisms of disease and therapeutic processes which would usually be impossible to obtain through clinical research. However, animal models do not necessarily behave in the same way as human patients. Studies in man, particularly the controlled clinical trials, are essential to the development of appropriate treatment. The practising clinician, however, deals with an individual patient and has to translate the findings from basic science research and large-scale multicentre trials into practical treatment.

Results from clinical trials cannot be directly translated into everyday clinical practice for various reasons. Strictly speaking, the trial results should be applicable only to the patient population who conform to the study inclusion and exclusion criteria. For instance, to apply the SAVE study results [1], it would be necessary for all patients to undergo radionuclide scintigraphy and exercise testing and, where appropriate, coronary bypass surgery or angioplasty before receiving captopril therapy after myocardial infarction. In practice, clinicians extrapolate from trial findings to their own patient population, and an inevitable part of practising medicine is the belief that the physicians are sufficiently knowledgeable of a particular trial to extrapolate appropriately.

Another aspect that needs to be highlighted is that some clinical trial results are more readily verified in clinical practice, for example, the efficacy of drugs in improving symptoms, although symptom scores are considered 'soft' endpoints. Results on survival cannot be verified in individual patients although mortality data are considered 'hard' endpoints. For instance, even though ACE inhibitors have been shown to improve survival of heart failure patients, the effects on symptoms and exercise capacity (i.e. markers of quality of life) are less certain [2]. It would be inappropriate to insist that a patient should persevere with unbearable cough or dizziness just because the physician believes that the drug will prolong his or her survival. The erosion of quality of life may amount to delaying death, rather than prolonging survival. Common-sense clinical judgement needs to be exercised. This requires a reasonable understanding of the trial results and their interpretation, and some idea of why the results were so, backed by an understanding of the mechanisms involved in the disease and therapeutic processes.

Selection of patients for ACE inhibitor therapy after myocardial infarction

The CONSENSUS II [3], Chinese, ISIS-4 and GISSI-3 [4] trials included patients with and without heart failure after acute myocardial infarction, whereas the SAVE [1], AIRE [5] and TRACE [6] studies included those with evidence of left ventricular dysfunction or heart failure. In other words, the latter patient populations are subsets of the former. The studies recruiting all patients then include those patients in SAVE, AIRE and TRACE, and there is overlap of patient groups between these latter three trials (Fig. 5.1).

From the available data so far, we can construct a table for comparison of the various trial results (Fig. 5.2). It is apparent that trials which include unselected patients post-myocardial infarction showed lower survival benefits that those which selected patients with cardiac dysfunction or failure. One explanation is a 'dilutional effect'. The

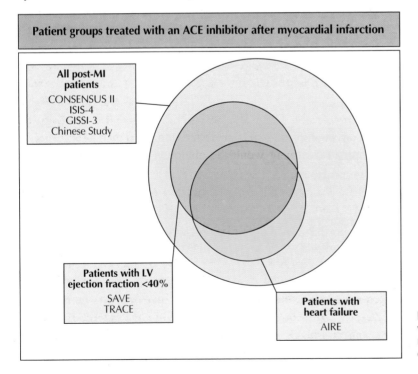

Fig. 5.1. Patient groups treated with an ACE inhibitor after myocardial infarction in the major clinical trials.

Number of deaths prevented or delayed with ACE inhibition after myocardial infarction		
Study	No. of 'lives saved'/1000 treated for first month	No. of 'lives saved'/1000 treated for first year
CONSENSUS II	0	0
ISIS-4	5	?
GISSI-3	8	?4
SAVE	?	?
AIRE	21	40

Fig. 5.2. The absolute numbers of deaths prevented or delayed reported in the main trials of ACE inhibitor therapy after acute myocardial infarction.

subgroup of patients with cardiac dysfunction or failure benefited markedly from the ACE inhibitor therapy, whereas the remainder derived little or no benefit and some may have been harmed [3,7], resulting in only marginal benefit in the trials of unselected patients.

Good clinical practice is essentially a balance between delivering benefits and minimizing harm. It appears from the trial results, therefore, that the judicious approach of introducing ACE-inhibitor therapy to appropriately selected patients is reasonable to adopt in practice. Patients who have severe damage to the ventricle after a myocardial infarction have a poor prognosis. Many will be receiving a diuretic and the need to start and continue ACE-inhibitor therapy is beyond question. More difficult is to decide how wide to make the indications for treatment with an ACE inhibitor. If these drugs had been convincingly shown to prevent reinfarction then justification for widespread treatment would be obvious. The limited evidence for such a benefit comes from post-hoc analysis in the SAVE study [8] with support from a similar analysis of the SOLVD data [9]. Short-term treatment in the GISSI-3 and ISIS-4 trials found no reduction in myocardial infarction [4]. Similarly, even with longer-term treatment, no reduction in myocardial infarction rate was seen in either CON-SENSUS II or the AIRE study [3,5]. Patients with cardiogenic shock should not be given ACE inhibitors but those in severe failure with adequate blood pressure seem likely to benefit. Previous infarction, old age, a large enzyme rise, especially with the pattern of an extensive antero-lateral myocardial infarction on the electrocardiogram would all be factors suggesting likely impairment of ventricular function and therefore particular benefit from ACE-inhibitor therapy. An objective estimate of ejection fraction or other measure of left ventricular function with the inherent limitations of such methods would further favour prescription of ACE inhibitors. The importance of clinical evidence of impaired ventricular function, however, in determining prognosis and benefit from ACE inhibition, irrespective of the ejection fraction, has been emphasized [10].

Patients thought not suitable for a beta blocker should in general be prescribed an ACE inhibitor. However, a substantial proportion could potentially benefit from both agents although some of their beneficial properties may overlap and their effects would not be additive. Careful monitoring of renal function is mandatory and particularly so in any patients receiving a potassium-sparing diuretic, steroid or anti-inflammatory drug other than low-dose aspirin.

Timing of introduction of ACE inhibitors

In the light of the results of the CONSENSUS-II trial (see Fig. 4.1), in which the mortality in the first 6 months was higher in the enalapril-treated group (although not statistically significant), and because the study was stopped prematurely because of 'statistical futility' and for reasons of safety [7], very early introduction of an ACE inhibitor after acute myocardial infarction (<24 hours using an intravenous route) should be avoided. The likely mechanisms of the harmful effects of such early introduction are discussed in Chapter 3. These include the potential ACE inhibitor-induced hypotension and impairment of the repair processes necessary after infarction. These repair processes are most important within the first few hours and days after infarction.

The authors of the GISSI-3 study write: "The strategy of early use of ACE inhibitors does not require an immediate decision but may be established on timely and careful observation of the haemodynamic status of the patients, during which the recommended treatments thrombolysis, aspirin and beta blockade are given, and glyceryl trinitrate is given when clinically indicated" [4]. Failure of ischaemic chest pain to resolve, low blood pressure and poor urine output, and complex arrhythmias, would make most clinicians delay starting ACE inhibitors after myocardial infarction.

The average times of introduction of ACE inhibitors in the SAVE and AIRE studies were 11 and 5–6 days after infarction, respectively [1,5]. Delayed introduction avoids the critical period of the post-infarct repair processes while maximizing the effects on the adverse remodelling processes which become progressive after the onset of cardiac failure. However, in the AIRE study substantial benefit on mortality was apparent within a short treatment period (30 days) and unnecessary delay seems therefore inappropriate. Furthermore, many patients die within the first 24–48 hours after infarction and fewer deaths, even though the differences were small, were found in this critical period in those receiving ACE inhibitors compared with those receiving placebo in the ISIS-4 study. No *a priori* reason was given, however, to anticipate a particular benefit in the first 24 hours. This observation should therefore be treated with some caution. What cannot be in doubt is the heterogeneity of patients after infarction; we regard the haemodynamic and ischaemic stability of the patient as a major influence in deciding whether to initiate ACE-inhibitor therapy. Our personal practice is to use intravenous nitrate therapy, which is easily controllable in the unstable situation, moving to ACE-inhibitor therapy after the first and often unpredictable 24 hours post-infarction period.

Which ACE inhibitor?

Are all ACE inhibitors the same? Inhibition of ACE is achieved by drugs that bind tightly to both of the enzyme's active sites, competitively blocking interactions between ACE and its two main substrates, angiotensin I and bradykinin. The potency and duration of action of each ACE inhibitor is largely determined by its physico-chemical and enzyme-kinetic characteristics. A broad categorization can be made according to whether the ACE inhibitor

- has a sulphydryl group (captopril and analogues)
- has a carboxyl group (enalapril and analogues)
- has a phosphorus group (fosinopril and analogues)

Many other features separate the different ACE inhibitors. These include tissue penetration, lipophilicity, substrate specificity, strong or weak bradykinin-potentiating effects, rapidity of absorption and onset of action, and duration of enzyme blockade. These are related, in part, to the broad structural classification.

The findings of the AIRE study [5] contrast markedly with those of SAVE [1]. Although both show clear mortality benefit in patients prescribed ACE inhibitors after myocardial infarction, the benefit was much more immediate and striking in AIRE than it was in SAVE. In

SAVE no separation of mortality curves was apparent until almost 1 year after beginning treatment, and subgroup analysis showed no definite survival benefit was apparent for the 40% of patients with clinical as well as radionuclide evidence of left ventricular dysfunction.

Different patient selection may account for these disparities but the properties of the individual ACE inhibitors cannot be discounted. Ramipril is a lipophilic prodrug containing a carboxyl group that binds avidly to ACE, producing long-lasting inhibition. Captopril is a hydrophilic drug containing a sulphydryl group that binds only weakly to ACE *in vivo* [11]. Differences in tissue distribution and extent of ACE inhibition seem likely in the two studies. Such issues will remain speculative unless comparative studies are performed.

What dose of ACE inhibitors should be used?

The recommended dosage and frequency of administration varies between clinical trials and relates predominantly to differences in the pharmacokinetic properties of the ACE inhibitors that have been studied.

The sulphydryl groups of captopril and its analogues act as strong zinc ligands. These drugs might therefore be expected to have both high potency and also long duration of action. *In vivo*, however, the length of action of captopril is limited by several reversible structural modifications (e.g. the formation of disulphide bonds) that occur as a result of interactions with endogenous sulphydryl-containing compounds. The carboxyl group of enalapril, ramipril and other analogues is a weak zinc ligand, but binds strongly to other parts of the ACE active sites. As a result, the carboxyl ACE inhibitors are generally more potent and have a longer duration of action than captopril. This allows less frequent administration of a lower dose. Fears that prolonged action could have disadvantages in patients with heart failure [12] have not been borne out in studies on many thousands of patients [5,13]. Nevertheless, short-acting ACE inhibitors could offer an advantage in the rare, severely salt-depleted individual patient.

The dosages of ACE inhibitor used in clinical trials differ considerably from those used in practice. Captopril, for example, was used at a target dose of 50 mg three time daily in SAVE [1] and twice daily in ISIS-4 [14], but is rarely used at such high doses in routine UK and

European practice. There is therefore concern that inappropriate dosages of this and other ACE inhibitors are often used [15]. Whether lower doses of ACE inhibitors confer the same beneficial survival effects is unknown. No study comparing high-dose and low-dose ACE inhibitors has been conducted.

Duration of ACE-inhibitor therapy after myocardial infarction

The ISIS-4 and GISSI-3 trials investigated the effects of short-term treatment (4–6 weeks) in all patients, irrespective of their risk of either progressive cardiac insufficiency or premature death. This strategy is based on the assumption that, as with thrombolytic therapy, early benefits are maintained long term irrespective of on-going therapy. It will be of interest to see whether initial small net benefits remain after 1 or more years. In the GISSI-3 study it is reported that the absolute mortality difference between drug and control group has halved by 6 months to 0.4% and is no longer significant [4].

In both the AIRE and SAVE studies treatment was continued indefinitely or until intolerance developed. The mortality curves continued to diverge throughout the follow-up period in both studies suggesting, although not proving, that long-term treatment had an on-going protective effect. However, on-going benefit would be in keeping with mechanistic considerations. For example, the occurrence of progressive ventricular dilatation in a subgroup of patients after acute myocardial infarction is said to indicate that cardiac insufficiency is also progressing [16]. ACE inhibitors seem able to attenuate this process, and the use of ACE-inhibitor therapy appears to produce most of its survival benefit by preventing deaths that have been preceded by worsening heart failure.

How long ACE-inhibitor therapy should continue is a question similar to that frequently posed concerning the use of beta blockers after myocardial infarction. Post-infarction patients are heterogenous; their natural history is varied. By 6 months after myocardial infarction, however, their prognosis is the same as any other group of similarly aged patients with ischaemic heart disease. The impact of the index infarction has waned markedly. Patients requiring diuretics for symptoms should continue therapy indefinitely whereas it would be difficult to justify continuing therapy in those observed to be asymptomatic with normal ejection fractions and normal ventricle sizes. Treatment of patients with reduced ejection fractions without symptoms remains contentious.

Monitoring treatment response

On an individual patient basis, it is impossible the determine whether ACE inhibition will enhance the patient's survival. We are far from knowing the exact mechanism by which ACE inhibition prolongs survival after myocardial infarction. Surrogate indicators have been proposed, such as ventricular dilatation, but, as has been discussed, dilatation *per se* may not be necessarily pathological or detrimental. Treating an individual patient for prognostic reasons is therefore essentially an act of faith which cannot be monitored.

There is little information on the impact of ACE inhibition following myocardial infarction on symptoms, functional capacity and other aspects of quality of life. Nevertheless, in attempting to prolong the life of patients, we should not compromise their quality of life. Constant attention should be paid to avoid serious adverse effects of therapy (see below). Other, less serious adverse effects, for example, cough, rash and non-specific reactions, may erode the quality of life sufficiently to necessitate withdrawal of ACE inhibitor therapy.

In chronic heart-failure patients, ACE inhibitor therapy does not consistently improve exercise tolerance [2]. With long-term treatment following myocardial infarction, however, we can expect better preservation of cardiac reserve assuming the hypothesis that ACE inhibition can reduce cardiac myocyte attrition rates without recurrence of infarction is correct [17,18]. This leads to both improved survival and preserved exercise capacity as assessed with cardiopulmonary exercise testing. Indeed, if ventricular dilatation were accompanied by improved exercise capacity, dilatation can be inferred as physiological.

Adverse effects of ACE inhibitors

The most important adverse reactions of ACE inhibition which need particular attention are renal dysfunction (especially in patients with overt or occult renal artery stenosis), electrolyte imbalance and hypotension.

Renal dysfunction

Patients with unilateral renal artery stenosis may undergo medical autonephrectomy without showing any significant deterioration in serum urea or creatinine. The most disastrous results are in the rare patients with bilateral renal artery stenoses where renal failure may be precipitated. However, in patients with poor cardiac output, lowering renal perfusion pressure further can also precipitate renal failure. The deterioration is reversible by stopping the ACE inhibitor and sometimes also the diuretic treatment but early detection of worsening renal function is essential. Daily monitoring of urea, creatinine and serum potassium is mandatory in high-risk patients, for example, those on high doses of diuretics, with already impaired renal function or with large falls in pressure on introduction of treatment. Less frequent monitoring is required for the majority. Levels of urea, creatinine and serum potassium should be measured before starting the ACE inhibitor and checked after 1 week with further checks at 1–3 monthly intervals. Deterioration in renal function is more important than absolute levels.

If the serum creatinine does not revert quickly to baseline values after cessation of ACE inhibition, then an urgent referral to a renal physician should be undertaken. It is worth remembering that the treatment of patients with heart failure is primarily dependent on their response to diuretics and, therefore, on reasonable renal function. Preservation of renal function is an important aim in treating heart failure. Particular care is needed where patients are taking steroid or non-steroidal anti-inflammatory agents.

Electrolyte imbalance

ACE inhibitors have a tendency to increase serum potassium, especially in patients with renal impairment. Careful balance with the dose of loop diuretics are necessary. There is no magic formula to obtain the ideal ratio of loop diuretics to ACE inhibitors. The only way to determine this is empirically, and this requires frequent checking of serum electrolytes. Combination with a potassium-sparing diuretic may be necessary (potassium supplements are not useful) to conserve both potassium and magnesium, but continued monitoring of serum potassium is obligatory. Heart-failure patients are prone to serious arrhythmias and sudden death; electrolyte imbalance is a factor inducing such arrhythmias. The majority of patients encounter no problem but the physician must remain vigilant to prevent harm to the minority.

Hypotension

ACE inhibitors are potent vasodilator agents. Patients with significant heart failure may not be able to tolerate the ensuing hypotension. Adjustment of the diuretic dose as well as of the ACE-inhibitor may, however, allow their use to continue in individual patients. Excessive hypotension, especially in the elderly patient, may result in detrimental consequences such as cerebral or myocardial ischaemia, resulting in falls or adverse cardiac sequelae. Supine and erect blood pressures should be regularly checked because postural hypotension, especially with loop diuretics, is quite common and may warn of impending problems which can be avoided by appropriate adjustment of the dose. The absolute blood pressure level has little relevance; it is the consequences, namely symptomatic hypotension or renal dysfunction, which require vigilance and appropriate action.

Conclusion

Thrombolytic agents are used to treat acute myocardial infarction, acting directly on the pathological process of coronary artery thrombosis. In contrast, the long-term treatment of patients with beta blockers represents a strategy of secondary prevention. Drugs such as aspirin have a role in both. It is therefore pertinent to consider into which of these two categories ACE inhibitors fall. Available data point to a mixed role, confirming treatment of heart failure together with prevention of deterioration in those with cardiac insufficiency.

Patients selected for treatment and secondary prevention on the basis of clinical manifestations of cardiac failure seem to benefit far more than those with reduced ejection fractions who are selected for secondary prevention alone. In contrast, patients without cardiac dysfunction have not yet been shown to derive either a treatment or a secondary-prevention benefit that is sufficient to justify routine use of an ACE inhibition.

Early administration of ACE inhibitors after myocardial infarction has the potential risk of introducing unnecessary harm in the form of hypotension and suppressing the compensatory and repair processes. On the other hand, their introduction should not be delayed unnecessarily. Once started, vigilant identification and treatment of adverse effects, especially careful monitoring of electrolytes and renal function, are essential to minimize harm in individual patients. Given that both the SAVE and AIRE trials show mortality curves which continue to diverge during the chronic phase of treatment, and the mechanistic possibility that ACE inhibition may reduce the on-going injurious effects of neurohormonal activation on the myocardium, it is reasonable to continue treatment long term.

References

1. Pfeffer MA, Braunwald E, Moyé LA, *et al.*: **Effect of captopril on mortality and morbidity in patients with left ventricular dysfunction after myocardial infarction. Results of the Survival and Ventricular Enlargement Trial.** *N Engl J Med* 1992, **327**:669–677.

2. Swedberg K, Gundersen T: **The role of exercise testing in heart failure.** *J Cardiovasc Pharmacol* 1993, **22** (suppl 9):S13–S17.

3. Swedberg K, Held P, Kjekshus J, Rasmussen K, Rydén L, Wedel H on behalf of the CONSENSUS II Study Group: **Effects of the early administration of enalapril on mortality in patients with acute myocardial infarction. Results of the Cooperative North Scandinavian Enalapril Survival Study II (CONSENSUS II).** *N Engl J Med* 1992, **327**:678–684.

4. Gruppo Italiano per lo Studio della Sopravvivenza nell'Infarto Miocardio: **GISSI-3 effects of lisinopril and transdermal glyceryl trinitrate singly and together on 6-week mortality and ventricular function after acute myocardial infarction.** *Lancet* 1994, **343**:1115–1122.

5. Acute Infarction Ramipril Efficacy (AIRE) Study Investigators: **Effects of ramipril on mortality and morbidity of survivors of acute myocardial infarction with clinical evidence of heart failure.** *Lancet* 1993, **342**:821–828.

6. The TRACE Study Group: **The TRAndopril Cardiac Evaluation (TRACE) Study: Rationale, design and baseline characteristics of the screened population.** *Am J Cardiol* 1994, **73**:44C–50C.

7. Furberg CD, Campbell RWF, Pi HB: **ACE inhibitors after myocardial infarction [letter].** *N Engl J Med* 1993, **328**:967–968.

8. Ganley CJ, Hung HMJ, Temple R: **More on the survival and ventricular enlargement trial.** *N Engl J Med* 1993, **329**:1204–1205.

9. Hall AS, Tan LB, Gray D, Ball SG: **ACE inhibitors for myocardial infarction and unstable angina.** *Lancet* 1992, **340**:1547.

10. Ball SG, Hall AS, Murray GD: **ACE inhibition, atherosclerosis and myocardial infarction – the AIRE study in practice.** *Eur Heart J* 1994, **15** (suppl B):20–25.

11. Unger T, Gohlike P: **Converting enzyme inhibitors in cardiovascular therapy: current status and future potential.** *Cardiovasc Res* 1994, **28**:146–158.

12. Cleland JGF, Dargie HJ, McAlpine H, *et al.*: **Severe hypotension after first dose of enalapril in heart failure.** *BMJ* 1985, **291**:1309–1314.

13. SOLVD Investigators: **Effects of enalapril on survival in patients with reduced left ventricular ejection fractions and congestive heart failure.** *N Engl J Med* 1991, **325**:293–302.

14. ISIS-4 Collaborative Group: **Fourth International Study of Infarct Survival: protocol for a large simple study of the effects of oral mononitrate, of oral captopril and of intravenous magnesium.** *Am J Cardiol* 1991, **68**:87D–100D.

15. Pouleur H: **High or low dose of angiotensin-converting enzyme inhibitor in patients with left ventricular dysfunction?** *Cardiovasc Drugs Ther* 1993, **7**:891–892.

16. Gaudron P, Eilles C, Ertl G, Kochsiek K: **Compensatory and noncompensatory left ventricular dilatation after myocardial infarction: time-course and haemodynamic consequences at rest and during exercise.** *Am Heart J* 1992, **123**:377–385.

17. Tan LB: **Clinical and research implications of new concepts in the assessment of cardiac pumping performance in heart failure.** *Cardiovasc Res* 1987, **21**:615–622.

18. Tan LB: **Evaluation of cardiac dysfunction, cardiac reserve and inotropic response.** *Postgrad Med J* 1991, **67** (suppl 1):S10–S20.

Index